D1609533

Teen Health Series

Stress Information For Teens, Second Edition

Stress Information For Teens, Second Edition

Health Tips About The Mental And Physical Consequences Of Stress

Including Facts About The Causes Of Stress, Types Of Stressors, Effects Of Stress, Strategies For Managing Stress, And More

Edited by Lisa Bakewell

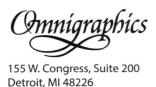

Omnigraphics

155 W. Congress, Suite 200
Detroit, MI 48226

Bibliographic Note

Because this page cannot legibly accommodate all the copyright notices, the Bibliographic Note portion of the Preface constitutes an extension of the copyright notice.

Edited by Lisa Bakewell

Teen Health Series

Karen Bellenir, *Managing Editor*
David A. Cooke, M.D., *Medical Consultant*
Elizabeth Collins, *Research and Permissions Coordinator*
EdIndex, *Services for Publishers, Indexers*

* * *

Omnigraphics, Inc.
Matthew P. Barbour, *Senior Vice President*
Kevin M. Hayes, *Operations Manager*

* * *

Peter E. Ruffner, *Publisher*
Copyright © 2014 Omnigraphics, Inc.
ISBN 978-0-7808-1315-1
E-ISBN 978-0-7808-1316-8

Library of Congress Cataloging-in-Publication Data

Stress information for teens : health tips about the mental and physical consequences of stress including information about the causes of stress, types of stressors, effects of stress, strategies for managing stress, and more / edited by Lisa Bakewell. -- Second edition.
     pages cm -- (Teen health series)
  Includes bibliographical references and index.
  Audience: Grade 9 to 12.
  Summary: "Provides basic consumer health information for teens about common causes of stress, the effects of stress on the body and mind, and coping strategies. Includes index, resource information, and recommendations for further reading"-- Provided by publisher.
  ISBN 978-0-7808-1315-1 (hardcover : alk. paper) 1. Stress management for teenagers. 2. Stress (Psychology) I. Bakewell, Lisa.
  RA785.S766 2013
  616.9'800835--dc23
                                                                    2013019169

Table of Contents

Part Three: Effects Of Stress On The Body, Mind, And Behavior

Part Four: Diseases And Disorders With A Possible Stress Component

Part Five: Stress Management

Part Six: If You Need More Information

Preface

About This Book

Most people go through times when they feel stressed out, but puberty's hormones can induce some especially confusing emotional and physical challenges in adolescents. The stresses teens feel can be good or bad. Some stress in response to internal or external pressures and expectations helps teens to perform well and motivates them to do their best. On the other hand, unrealistic or overwhelming pressure stops being helpful, and it can have a negative impact on teens' health, mood, productivity, relationships, and behavior. Furthermore, stress left unchecked may result in emotional and physical consequences that can last a lifetime.

Stress Information For Teens, Second Edition helps readers understand what stress is, recognize the different types of stressors, and realize how stress affects the adolescent mind, body, and behavior. Common causes of teen stress are discussed, and diseases and disorders having possible stress components (including asthma, back pain, chronic fatigue, peptic ulcers, eczema, hair loss, and eating disorders) are explained. Facts about successful practices, therapies, and techniques for handling anger, improving body image and self-esteem, and relieving stress (such as exercise, relaxation techniques, massage therapy, meditation, yoga, art therapies, pet interaction, and journaling) are also included. The book concludes with a directory of stress and stress management resources and suggestions for additional reading.

How To Use This Book

This book is divided into parts and chapters. Parts focus on broad areas of interest; chapters are devoted to single topics within a part.

Part One: Understanding Stress explains the distinctions between acute stress (short-term) and chronic stress (long-term), gender-related differences in stress responses, and age-related factors involved in distinguishing between danger and safety. It also discusses how suitable reactions to potentially stressful situations can actually help build resilience and self-esteem.

Part Two: Common Causes Of Stress In Teens includes information about the most frequent sources of stress among adolescents, including test anxiety, peer pressure, friendship issues, dating concerns, overbooked schedules, and sports competition. It also discusses stressors related to family life experiences (such as financial difficulty, violence, substance abuse, and divorce), current events, and social anxieties. In addition, the causes and consequences of bullying—in person and online (cyberbullying)—are addressed.

Part Three: Effects Of Stress On The Body, Mind, And Behavior describes the various ways childhood stress can reach across the entire lifespan. It discusses how stress affects the immune system, the potential link between stress and cancer, and how stress can change the brain—both physically and psychologically. Stress-related mental and behavioral disorders are addressed, including eating disorders, body dysmorphic disorder, self-injury, depression, and suicide. The special concerns associated with stresses related to loss and grief are also discussed.

Part Four: Diseases And Disorders With A Possible Stress Component explores how some illness and other health issues might be stress related. Chapters with information on medical conditions linked to stress triggers, such as asthma, chronic fatigue syndrome, fibromyalgia, multiple sclerosis, lupus, peptic ulcers, chronic heartburn, and bowel syndromes, are included. Also, physical manifestations of chronic stress, including back pain, eczema, and hair loss, are discussed.

Part Five: Stress Management provides information on stress reduction techniques, including exercise, meditation, and relaxation. It discusses how laughter, spirituality, journaling, pets, and art therapies can be used to help relieve stress and how talking to parents, therapists, and other adults has the potential to offer additional health benefits. In addition, the importance of anger management is addressed.

Part Six: If You Need More Information includes suggestions for additional reading and a directory of organizations able to provide further materials about adolescent stress.

Bibliographic Note

This volume contains documents and excerpts from publications issued by the following government agencies: Center for Disease Control and Prevention (CDC); National Cancer Institute; National Center for Complementary and Alternative Medicine; National Institute on Alcohol Abuse and Alcoholism; National Institute of Allergy and Infectious Diseases; National Institute of Arthritis and Musculoskeletal and Skin Diseases; National Institute of Diabetes and Digestive and Kidney Diseases; National Institutes of Health; National Institute of Mental Health; National Institute of Neurological Disorders and Stroke; National Science Foundation; Office on Women's Health; StopBullying.gov; Substance Abuse and Mental Health Services Administration; U.S. Department of Health and Human Services; and the U.S. Department of Veterans Affairs.

In addition, this volume contains copyrighted documents and articles produced by the following organizations and individuals: A.D.A.M., Inc.; About.com; American Psychological Association; Better Health Channel, State Government of Victoria (Australia); Center for Young Women's Health; Cleveland Clinic Foundation; Government of Newfoundland and Labrador (Canada); Helpguide; Maternal and Family Health Services; Michigan Department of Corrections; Montana Attorney General, Montana Department of Justice; National Eczema Society; National Multiple Sclerosis Society; Nemours Foundation; North American Spine Society; Palo Alto Medical Foundation; Pennsylvania Department of Health, Phoenix House; PsychCentral; Elizabeth Scott; Students Against Destructive Decisions (SADD); and Women's and Children's Health Network.

The photograph on the front cover is © iStockphoto via Thinkstock (www.thinkstock photos.com).

Full citation information is provided on the first page of each chapter. Every effort has been made to secure all necessary rights to reprint the copyrighted material. If any omissions have been made, please contact Omnigraphics to make corrections for future editions.

Acknowledgements

In addition to the organizations listed above, special thanks are due to Bonnie L. Stafford, best cheerleader ever; Liz Collins, research and permissions coordinator; Karen Bellenir, managing editor; and WhimsyInk, prepress services provider.

About The *Teen Health Series*

At the request of librarians serving today's young adults, the *Teen Health Series* was developed as a specially focused set of volumes within Omnigraphics' *Health Reference Series*. Each volume deals comprehensively with a topic selected according to the needs and interests of people in middle school and high school.

Teens seeking preventive guidance, information about disease warning signs, medical statistics, and risk factors for health problems will find answers to their questions in the *Teen Health Series*. The *Series*, however, is not intended to serve as a tool for diagnosing illness, in prescribing treatments, or as a substitute for the physician/patient relationship. All people concerned about medical symptoms or the possibility of disease are encouraged to seek professional care from an appropriate health care provider.

If there is a topic you would like to see addressed in a future volume of the *Teen Health Series*, please write to:

Editor
Teen Health Series
Omnigraphics, Inc.
155 West Congress, Suite 200
Detroit, MI 48226

A Note About Spelling And Style

Teen Health Series editors use *Stedman's Medical Dictionary* as an authority for questions related to the spelling of medical terms and the *Chicago Manual of Style* for questions related to grammatical structures, punctuation, and other editorial concerns. Consistent adherence is not always possible, however, because the individual volumes within the *Series* include many documents from a wide variety of different producers and copyright holders, and the editor's primary goal is to present material from each source as accurately as is possible following the terms specified by each document's producer. This sometimes means that information in different chapters or sections may follow other guidelines and alternate spelling authorities. For example, occasionally a copyright holder may require that eponymous terms be shown in possessive forms (Crohn's disease *vs.* Crohn disease) or that British spelling norms be retained (leukaemia *vs.* leukemia).

Locating Information Within The *Teen Health Series*

The *Teen Health Series* contains a wealth of information about a wide variety of medical topics. As the *Series* continues to grow in size and scope, locating the precise information needed by a specific student may become more challenging. To address this concern, information about books within the *Teen Health Series* is included in *A Contents Guide to the Health Reference Series*. The *Contents Guide* presents an extensive list of more than 16,000 diseases, treatments, and other topics of general interest compiled from the Tables of Contents and major index headings from the books of the *Teen Health Series* and *Health Reference Series*. To access *A Contents Guide to the Health Reference Series*, visit www.healthreferenceseries.com.

Our Advisory Board

We would like to thank the following advisory board members for providing guidance to the development of this *Series*:

Dr. Lynda Baker, Associate Professor of Library and Information Science, Wayne State University, Detroit, MI

Medical Consultant

Medical consultation services are provided to the *Teen Health Series* editors by David A. Cooke, MD. Dr. Cooke is a graduate of Brandeis University, and he received his MD degree from the University of Michigan. He completed residency training at the University of Wisconsin Hospital and Clinics. He is board-certified in internal medicine. Dr. Cooke currently works as part of the University of Michigan Health System and practices in Ann Arbor, MI. In his free time, he enjoys writing, science fiction, and spending time with his family.

Part One
Understanding Stress

Chapter 1

What Is Stress?

Stress is the emotional and physical strain caused by the response to pressure from the outside world. Unfortunately, there is no universally agreed upon definition of stress, and individuals react differently to stress. What is stressful for one person may be pleasurable or have little effect on others. Stress is not necessarily bad; in small doses, it can help people perform under pressure and motivate them to do their best. But, beyond a certain point, stress stops being helpful and starts causing damage to health, mood, productivity, relationships, and quality of life.

Stress is a normal physical response to events that make a person feel threatened or upset. When danger is sensed—whether it is real or imagined—the body's defenses kick into high gear in a rapid, automatic process known as the fight-or-flight reaction, or the stress response. The brain signals the release of stress hormones. These chemical substances trigger a series of responses that gives the body extra energy: blood sugar levels rise, the heartbeat speeds up, and blood pressure increases. The muscles tense for action. The blood supply is diverted away from the core to the extremities to help the body deal with the situation at hand. The stress response is the body's way of protecting itself.

Are there different types of stress?

Stress management can be complicated and confusing because there are different types of stress: acute stress, episodic acute stress, chronic stress, and posttraumatic stress, each with its own characteristics, symptoms, duration, and treatment approaches.

About This Chapter: Information in this chapter is excerpted from "Stress and Stress Management," from the Substance Abuse and Mental Health Services Administration (www.samhsa.gov), March 2009, U.S. Department of Health and Human Services.

- **Acute Stress:** The most common form of stress is acute stress. It comes from demands and pressures of the recent past and anticipated demands and pressures of the near future. Because it is short-term, acute stress does not have enough time to do the extensive damage associated with long-term stress. Acute stress can crop up in anyone's life, and it is highly treatable and manageable.

- **Episodic Acute Stress:** Those who suffer acute stress frequently are dealing with episodic acute stress. It is common for people with episodic acute stress to be over-aroused, short-tempered, irritable, anxious, and tense. Interpersonal relationships deteriorate rapidly when others respond with real hostility. Work becomes a very stressful place for them. Often, lifestyle and personality issues are so ingrained and habitual with these individuals that they see nothing wrong with the way they conduct their lives. They blame their woes on other people and external events. Frequently, they see their lifestyles, patterns of interacting with others, and ways of perceiving the world as part and parcel of who and what they are. Without proper coping strategies, episodic acute stress develops into chronic stress.

- **Chronic Stress:** The grinding stress that wears people away day after day, year after year is called chronic stress. It destroys bodies, minds, and lives. It is the stress of unrelenting demands and pressures for seemingly interminable periods of time. The worst aspect of chronic stress is that people get used to it. They forget it is there. People are immediately aware of acute stress because it is new. Chronic stress is ignored because it is familiar and almost comfortable.

- **Posttraumatic Stress Disorder (PTSD):** PTSD stems from traumatic experiences that become internalized and remain forever painful and present. Individuals experiencing PTSD could exhibit signs of hyper vigilance (an easily triggered startle response). People with an exaggerated startle response are easily startled by any number of things (e.g., loud noises, doors slamming, shouting). They usually feel tense or on edge. Along with hyper vigilance, people experiencing PTSD symptoms also could be dealing with avoidance issues—including staying away from places, events, or objects that are reminders of the experience; feeling emotionally numb; feeling strong guilt, depression, or worry; losing interest in activities that were enjoyable in the past; and having trouble remembering the dangerous event. People experiencing PTSD symptoms wear down to breaking points because physical and mental resources are depleted through long-term attrition. The symptoms of posttraumatic stress are difficult to treat and may require the help of a doctor or mental health professional.

How does stress affect people?

Stress is taking a toll on people—contributing to health problems, poor relationships, and lost productivity at work, according to a national survey released by the American Psychological Association (APA). Twenty-eight percent of Americans say that they are managing their stress extremely well. However, many people report experiencing physical symptoms (77 percent) and psychological symptoms (73 percent) related to stress. While Americans deal with high levels of stress on a daily basis, the health consequences are most serious when that stress is poorly managed. The body does not distinguish between physical and psychological threats. Everyone reacts differently to stress, and each body sends out a different set of red flags.

Common Myths Surrounding Stress

- **Myth: Stress is the same for everyone.** In fact, stress is different for everyone. What is stressful for one person may or may not be stressful for another. Each person may respond to stress in an entirely different way.

- **Myth: Stress is always bad.** According to this view, zero stress makes us happy and healthy. This is wrong—stress is a normal part of life. Stress can be the kiss of death or the spice of life. The issue is how to manage it. Managed stress makes people productive and happy. Mismanaged stress hurts and even kills.

- **Myth: Stress is everywhere, so nothing can be done about it.** Not so. Life can be planned so that stress does not become overwhelming.

- **Myth: The most popular techniques for reducing stress are the best ones.** Actually, no universally effective stress reduction techniques exist because each individual reacts differently.

- **Myth: No symptoms, no stress.** Absence of symptoms does not mean the absence of stress. In fact, camouflaging symptoms with medication may deprive a person of the signals needed for reducing the strain on physiological and psychological systems.

- **Myth: Only major symptoms of stress require attention.** This myth assumes that minor symptoms, such as headaches or stomach acid, may be safely ignored. Minor symptoms of stress are the early warnings that life is getting out of hand and stress needs to be better managed.

Source: Information adapted from American Psychological Association, 2008, and excerpted from "Stress and Stress Management," Substance Abuse and Mental Health Services Administration, March 2009.

Is stress experienced differently by genders or generations?

The APA reported that nearly half of Americans state that their stress levels have increased since November 2007, with as many as 30 percent rating their average stress levels as extreme (eight, nine, or 10—on a 10-point scale—where 10 means "a great deal of stress"). At the same time, economic conditions take a physical and emotional toll on people nationwide. Compared with men, more women say they are stressed about the following issues:

- Money (83 percent vs. 78 percent)
- The economy (84 percent vs. 75 percent)
- Housing costs (66 percent vs. 58 percent)
- Health problems affecting their families (70 percent vs. 63 percent)

Across the board, women are reporting higher levels of stress, are more likely than men to cite various stressors, and report more physical and emotional symptoms as a result of stress, suggesting that stress is having a significant impact on women.

In reports released by the APA, older adults report having less stress and managing stress better than younger adults, however, the financial crisis is having a greater impact on older generations—leading to more stress at work. Many older adults are waiting to retire or coming out of retirement and joining the workforce to make ends meet.

Does stress look different across cultures?

Stress is common to all people regardless of ethnicity. However, sources of stress vary among cultural groups. All cultural groups are reporting increased stress about money and work. However, as a result of cultural norms, many ethnic groups are having difficulty asking for help regarding coping skills. When it comes to managing stress, the APA reports that several cultural groups say they are doing enough to manage their stress; however, groups do not report that they are managing their stress well. It is important to maintain a sense of identity and social support when feeling overwhelmed and stressed. This includes embracing cultural background when developing a personal strategy for dealing with stress.

What are the warning signs of stress?

It is important to learn how to recognize when stress levels are dangerously high. The most dangerous thing about stress is how easily it can get out of control. Many factors can cause it, but common triggers tend to be the pressures of work, relationships, money, or family problems, or merely the fact that life suddenly seems to be a constant tough battle. One of the important aids for combating and dealing with stress is to first recognize it. Stress affects minds, bodies, and behaviors in many ways, and everyone experiences stress differently. A body's stress warning signs alert a person that something is not right, much like the glowing "check engine" light on a car's dashboard.

Can stress be prevented?

Stressful situations in life cannot be prevented. However, they can be prepared for in a way that allows a positive response. This is done by building and fostering resilience in different areas of life. Resilience implies that after an event, a person or community may not only be able to cope and recover, but also change to reflect different priorities arising from the experience and prepare for the next stressful situation. Fostering resilience, or the ability to bounce back from a stressful situation, builds a proactive mechanism to manage stress. Developing a greater level of resilience will not prevent stressful conditions from happening, but it can reduce the level of disruption a stressor has and the time it takes to recover.

How can stress be managed?

Stress can be dealt with proactively or reactively. It can be dealt with proactively by building personal resilience to prepare for stressful circumstances, while learning how to recognize signs and symptoms of stress. It can be dealt with reactively by utilizing coping strategies useful for the individual. The key is not to avoid stress altogether, but to manage the stress in such a way that the negative consequences of stress are avoided. There are many positive ways to manage stress.

The best defense against stress is building resilience. Resilience refers to the ability of an individual, family, organization, or community to cope with adversity and adapt to challenges

Common Stressors

- Financial issues: 81 percent of Americans worry about this topic
- Work and job stability: 67 percent of Americans worry about this topic
- The Nation's economy: 80 percent of Americans worry about this topic
- Health concerns (family and personal): 64 percent of Americans worry about this topic
- Relationships: 62 percent of Americans worry about this topic
- Personal safety: 48 percent of Americans worry about this topic
- Loss: 72 percent of Americans worry about this topic

Source: Data from American Psychological Association, 2008, and excerpted from "Stress and Stress Management," Substance Abuse and Mental Health Services Administration, March 2009.

or change. It is a process of drawing on beliefs, behaviors, skills, and attitudes to move beyond stress, trauma, or tragedy. While building defenses through resilience, it also is important to be ready to deal with stress if the internal resilience reservoir is not enough.

Managing stress can include simple ideas, such as recognizing signs of stress, learning breathing techniques, and engaging in spiritual communities, and more advanced interventions with professionals, such as seeking the help of a mental health professional and learning stress inoculation techniques. The goal of stress inoculation is to develop a procedure that will almost instantaneously put a person in a calm state. This is not necessarily a completely relaxed condition since many demanding situations will not allow that. The idea, however, is to be able to step back and look at problematic circumstances in a realistic light without feeling too hassled.

Uncontrolled stress can lead to many problems. Simple headaches, tight muscles, problems with sleeping, or a bad mood can be a prelude to much more severe symptoms. There are many healthy ways to manage and cope with stress, but they all require change: either changing the situation or changing reactions to the situation. If stress is affecting a person's ability to work or find pleasure in life, help should be sought from a doctor, mental health provider, or other professional.

Warning Signs Of Stress

Cognitive Signs
- Memory problems
- Inability to concentrate
- Poor judgment
- Negativity
- Anxious or racing thoughts
- Constant worrying

Emotional Signs
- Moodiness
- Irritability or short temper
- Agitation, inability to relax
- Feeling overwhelmed
- Sense of loneliness and isolation
- Depression or general unhappiness

Physical Signs
- Aches and pains
- Headaches
- Diarrhea or constipation
- Nausea, dizziness
- Chest pain, rapid heartbeat
- Loss of sex drive
- Frequent colds

Behavioral Signs
- Eating more or less
- Sleeping too much or too little
- Isolating from others
- Procrastinating or neglecting responsibilities
- Using alcohol, cigarettes, or drugs to relax
- Nervous habits (e.g., nail biting, pacing)

Source: Information adapted from Mental Health America, 2007, and excerpted from "Stress and Stress Management," Substance Abuse and Mental Health Services Administration, March 2009.

Chapter 2

Short- And Long-Term Stress

What Is Short-Term Stress?

Have you ever started a new school, argued with your best friend, or moved? Do you have to deal with the ups and downs of daily life—like homework or your parents' expectations? Then you already know about stress. In fact, everyone experiences stress. Your body is pre-wired to deal with it—whether it is expected or not. This response is known as the stress response, or fight or flight.

The fight or flight response is as old as the hills. In fact, when people used to have to fight off wild animals to survive, fight or flight is what helped them do it. Today, different things cause stress (when was the last time you had to fend off a grizzly bear?), but we still go through fight or flight. It prepares us for quick action, which is why the feeling goes away once whatever was stressing you out passes! It can also happen when something major happens—like if you change schools or have a death in your family.

Everyone has weird feelings when they are stressed. Fight or flight can cause things like sweaty palms or a dry mouth when you are nervous, or knots in your stomach after an argument with someone. This is totally normal and means that your body is working exactly like it should. There are lots of signs of stress—common types are physical (butterflies in your stomach), emotional (feeling sad or worried), behavioral (you don't feel like doing things), and mental (you can't concentrate). Most physical signs of stress usually don't last that long and can help you perform better, if you manage them right.

About This Chapter: The information in this chapter is excerpted from "Got Butterflies? Find Out Why," Centers for Disease Control and Prevention (www.bam.gov), January 2013.

So, when you feel stress, what happens to make your body do the things it does? According to the experts, three glands "go into gear" and work together to help you cope with change or a stressful situation. Two are in your brain and are called the hypothalamus (hipe-o-thal-a-mus) and the pituitary (pi-to-i-tary) gland. The third, the adrenal (a-dree-nal) glands, are on top of your kidneys. The hypothalamus signals your pituitary gland that it is time to tell your adrenal glands to release the stress hormones called epinephrine (ep-in-efrin), norepinenphrine (nor-ep-in-efrin), and cortisol (cor-ti-sol). These chemicals increase your heart rate and breathing and provide a burst of energy—which is useful if you're trying to run away from a bear! These chemicals can also control body temperature (which can make you feel hot or cold), keep you from getting hungry, and make you less sensitive to pain. Because everyone is different, everyone will have different signs. Not to worry—everyone experiences these physical signs of stress sometimes. The good news is that, once things return to normal, your body will turn off the stress response. After some rest and relaxation, you'll be good as new. Following are examples of short-term stress.

Cold Hands/Dry Mouth/Pounding Heart

- You're about to take a big test or star in the school play and you've got cold hands, a mouth as dry as the desert, and your heart is pounding.

Cold Hands

Because you're nervous and under pressure to perform, your body has kicked the stress response into high gear. The stress hormones are shooting through your bloodstream and moving your blood away from your skin. This can give your heart and muscles more strength—which you would really need if you were trying to run away. Because your blood is going to the places that really need it (like your heart, lungs, and liver), your hands can be left feeling like ice.

Dry Mouth

Once that stress response is running full force, your body sends your blood to only those parts that are truly necessary for you to survive. Lots of the fluid in your body goes to really important places (like your organs) and can leave you with a mouth as dry as the desert. Because your blood is busy with your organs and not your muscles, your throat (which is made of muscle) can tighten, making it hard to swallow.

Pounding Heart

When you're starring in the school play, your body wants to give you what you need to succeed—which goes back to the fight or flight response. Your heart will start pounding to help you out! In fact, it is one of the first signs of the stress response. It happens because the release of stress hormones can speed up the flow of your blood by 300–400 percent! Your heart has to beat much faster to move all of that blood to your organs and your muscles. This provides a burst of energy that can help you get through backstage jitters and the first few minutes of your play.

Everyone experiences stress. If you have any of these signs of stress, it means that your body is doing its job. Try to relax and check this out for some easy ways to cope with stress.

Red Face/Lots Of Sweat

- You're about to make an election speech for student council and your face is beet red, and you are sweaty all over.

Even though it's just a speech and you aren't planning on fighting off any tigers, remember what you are feeling is part of the fight or flight response. The body turns on its climate control system, raises its temperature, and produces sweat—and lots of it. Originally, this helped your body cool in case you did need to run away from a horde of wild animals. Of course, now that your making your speech (which is the modern day equivalent of facing down those tigers and bears), you end up drenched in sweat and your face is the color of a fire engine.

Butterflies/Knots

- It's your first day back at school, or maybe you're starting a new school, and you've got butterflies in your stomach.

Stomachaches, or a queasy feeling, happen all the time in stressful situations like this. And it's no wonder. Once the stress response kicks into high gear, one of the stress hormones (cortisol) shuts the stomach down and won't let food digest. It can also put your digestive tract into high speed, making you feel nauseated.

Can't Concentrate?

- You have so much to do, but you just can't seem to concentrate.

Got too much to do? You know how it goes—you have tons of homework to do RIGHT NOW, you've got a game this afternoon, your little brother is annoying you, and your mom is insisting that you clean your room—but you just can't seem to focus on any one thing. You feel like you have no energy to finish all that you've got to do. This is because the stress hormones fill up your short-term memory with the immediate demands of dealing with stress. They also signal your brain to store the memory of the stressful event in your long-term memory so you know how to respond the next time something stressful happens. All of this means you are more likely to forget something, feel like you can't concentrate, snap at your family, be mean to a friend, or feel tongue-tied.

What Is Long-Term Stress?

But what happens when life continues to throw curves at you and if you have one stressful event after another? Your stress response may not be able to stop itself from running overtime,

Stress, A Positive Life Force

Stress is a basic force of life which can allow us to reach higher levels of performance. Regardless of whether pleasant or unpleasant events cause the stress, when managed properly, stress can be a powerful ally for growth and accomplishment.

Without stress, our lives would be monotonous. Stress is the automatic state that results when the body is told to make changes in order to adapt to any demand.

There are two types of stress. The first kind is eustress, which is the "good" kind of stress. This type keeps us challenged and is necessary for effective performance to achieve certain goals. Eustress, or "good" stress, helps us accomplish things. It gets our adrenaline going by forcing us to set deadlines, goals, or take action. For example, an athlete enjoys lifting the heavier weights because the sensation of sore muscles means that they are becoming stronger and more toned. Stress for an athlete means expending more energy to fulfill his or her dreams of breaking new records, and performing on demand at full potential.

The second kind of stress is distress. Distress is the "unpleasant" kind. This stress requires us to constantly readjust or adapt to a major change or traumatic situation. Examples of distress are death of a family member, family financial problems, or your parents' divorce.

Stress affects each of us differently depending on the meaning we place on various events and how we think about them. In order for stress to be a positive force in our lives, we should focus on what we can do to help minimize its negative effects. You can begin this process with a simple inventory.

1. **Identify what's stressful to you.** Different people react to similar stressors in different ways. What may be stressful to one person may not be stressful to you.

2. **Identify how stress affects you.** Do you feel anxious, worry more than usual, feel depressed, have mood swings, experience difficulty sleeping, feel agitated, have headaches, upset stomach or feel fatigue? To handle stress in a more healthy way, we can either eliminate the source of distress or find out how to manage the stress.

3. **Identify when you are most vulnerable to stress.** Identify the time of day, week, or a certain time of the month (or year) that you feel more stressed.

and you may not have a chance to rest, restore, and recuperate. This can add up and, suddenly, the signs of overload hit you—turning short-term stressors into long-term stress. This means that you may have even more physical signs of stress. Things like a headache, eating too much or not at all, tossing and turning all night, or feeling down and angry all the time, are all signs of long-term stress. These signs start when you just can't deal with any more.

Long-term stress can affect your health and how you feel about yourself, so it is important to learn to deal with it. No one is completely free of stress and different people respond to it

4. **Identify when stress is good for you.** Stress can be one of our best defense mechanisms. For example, if we sense that we are in danger of an automobile hitting us, our bodies can respond by releasing adrenaline and other chemicals that can increase our alertness, raise blood pressure, increase strength, speed, and our reaction time to help us get out of the way of an oncoming motor vehicle.

5. **Identify how you manage your stress.** The goal is to be able to manage your stress rather than to try to eliminate it. There will always be some stress in our lives and to best cope, we need to be able to identify the stressors, and understand the feelings the stressors generate.

6. **Take advantage of strategies to manage stress**. Small changes over time can have a tremendous impact on our body's ability to fight off the negative impacts of stress.

A stressor is not the same as stress. The stressor is any physical or non-physical event that caused the stress reaction or feeling. You can choose your attitude. You decide if it is a positive or a negative one. Effective stress management combines a healthy lifestyle, management of emotions, and the ability to think differently. Here are some effective ways to cope with stress:

- Decrease/limit caffeine intake.
- Set goals.
- Don't use alcohol or drugs as stress reducers.
- Get at least seven to eight hours of sleep every 24 hours.
- Eat a nourishing breakfast.
- Eat more fruits, vegetables, salads, whole grain breads, egg whites, and meats that are broiled or grilled.
- Learn skills to improve work and/or personal relationships.
- Include fun and pleasure in your life with humor, music, or a hobby.
- Don't sweat the small stuff.
- Consult your physician or personal trainer about an exercise program.

Source: Information in this box is excerpted from "Stress, A Positive Life Force," November 2004, © 2004 State of Michigan. Reprinted with permission from the Michigan Department of Corrections (http://www.michigan.gov/corrections). Information in this box has been reviewed by David A. Cooke, MD, FACP, April 2013.

in lots of different ways. The most important thing to learn about long-term stress is how to spot it. You can do that by listening to your body signals and learning healthy ways to handle it. Following are examples of possible symptoms of long-term stress.

Headache

- It's been a long, tense day and you feel like you've got a rubber band squeezing around your head that just won't stop.

Headaches are one of the most common signs of long-term stress. They can feel dull and achy—just like a rubber band tightening around your head. Although it is unclear what exactly causes these headaches, tight head and neck muscles are generally thought to be to blame. The chemical messengers in your brain get really busy and tell your blood vessels to get really small. This means that less blood is getting to your head—and that can cause a headache. Your eyes, forehead, or the top of your head will be the first places you feel the pain.

Sleeplessness

- You're exhausted but when you try to sleep, you lie awake for hours.

During the day, the levels of hormones that give you energy (epinephrine and norepinephrine) and those that help you stay happy (called dopamine) stay consistent. Towards the end of a normal day, these hormones begin to decrease and the hormone that helps you sleep (called serotonin) kicks into high gear. But if you've been trapped in a stress cycle, your body continues to produce those stress hormones from the adrenal glands. They "rev" up your body and block out the serotonin, making it hard to sleep even if you feel tired.

Change In Appetite

- You've just had a fight with your best friend and eating is the only thing that makes you feel better—or maybe you feel like you could never eat again.

While you might become ravenous after a stressful event, your best friend might be grossed out by the thought of food. It just depends on how your body reacts to stress. If you get hungry, you may crave comfort foods (like candy bars, soda, or ice cream) because they increase the levels of a feel-good hormone called serotonin in the body—meaning that you will be in a better mood. Keep in mind that your body is just responding to the stress you are feeling and that your appetite will go back to normal.

14

On the other hand, your best friend might lose her appetite because the stress hormones make it difficult for her to eat. If you can't eat when you're stressed, try something small—like peanut butter on toast or a piece of fruit.

Overwhelmed?

- You are starting to feel overwhelmed by it all and you don't know if you can handle it.

Everyone has different ideas of what you should be doing and it feels like you have so many different roles to play—good student, kid, brother, sister, and friend—that things can sometimes seem out of control. It can make you tired just thinking about all you have to do! If you're feeling overwhelmed, you may notice that you can't sleep—which makes you tired and cranky. Then, you realize that you don't feel like doing the things you like to do and you feel a little bit sad or anxious. You may begin to feel achy and tired all over. These are signs of being stressed out. Your stress response system is having a hard time turning off. Don't panic—your body is just trying to tell you something. Take the time to figure out what is stressing you out and try to lessen the load you're carrying.

Anger

- Things are crazy right now, and you just don't have any patience with anyone. You feel angry at someone at the drop of a hat.

Anger is another common response to stress. Often, people who have been locked into a stress cycle feel helpless and overwhelmed. Once this happens, they can get angry much more quickly and they lash out at anyone that gets in their way. In fact, everyone at one point or another gets angry because they are stressed out.

Chapter 3

Adolescents And Stress

Teen Brain More Vulnerable To Stress

Teen brains rely on early-maturing brain structures that process fear differently than adult brains, according to study funded by the National Institute of Mental Health (NIMH). As a result, teens may have more difficulty than adults in differentiating between danger and safety, leading to more pervasive stress and anxiety.

Background

Things that frighten children or teens generally no longer frighten them as adults. So how does the adult brain distinguish between danger and safety, and what does the developing brain do differently?

To explore these questions, Jennifer Lau, PhD, of Oxford University (formerly at NIMH), and colleagues compared the brain activity of healthy youth with healthy adults during a threat learning task. In this task, participants were shown a series of photos that showed:

- A person with a neutral expression at first, then a fearful expression paired with a loud scream; or, in some later photos, the same person with a neutral expression only (threat stimulus)

- A different person with a neutral expression only (safety stimulus)

Immediately after each photo, participants rated how afraid they felt.

About This Chapter: The information in this chapter is excerpted from "Teen Brain Less Discerning of Threat vs. Safety, More Vulnerable to Stress," National Institute of Mental Health (www.nimh.nih.gov), April 2011.

Teens And Stress

Stressing out about a boyfriend or girlfriend or history test is part of a typical day for a teenager. But what is making these insignificant events seem like the end of the world?

With help from the National Science Foundation (NSF), Adriana Galván, a psychologist at the University of California, Los Angeles (UCLA), has been studying the effects of stress on teenagers and adults.

"Teenagers experience stress as more stressful," says Galván, "and if that stress is interfering with their decision making, it's really important to understand the neural mechanism that's underlying this connection between high levels of stress and poor decision making."

Galván's ground-breaking study focuses on the effect stress has on brain function. Study participants report their stress level daily, using a one to seven scale—seven being the worst. If participants rate their day as a seven, Galván will ask them to visit the lab for tests.

Nilufer Rustomji, an 18-year-old participant of the study, rates her day's stress level as a seven. Monitoring her brain function with Magnetic Resonance Imaging (MRI), Galván asks Rustomji to play a simple "reward and risk" video game, which involves wagering money.

"During the game, Rustomji is evaluating risk," explains Galván, "and while she's doing that evaluation, we are taking pictures of the brain to see how the brain makes [such] risky choices."

After computer processing the images, Galván analyzes how stress and risk influence what she calls the "reward system."

"The teenagers show more activation in the reward system than adults when making risky choices, and they are also making more risky choices than adults are," says Galván.

The prefrontal cortex is the part of the brain that helps regulate behavior but in adolescents, this region is not fully developed.

To help lower teens' stress, Galván says teens should double check and think about how the consequences will affect them later. "When you are stressed out as a teenager, it's interfering with your ability to make decisions," says Galván. "It's interfering with how the brain functions in regions that are still developing, mainly the reward system and the prefrontal cortex."

Galván's study is helping to provide deeper insight into why teenagers often act the way they do.

Source: The information in this box is excerpted from "Teens and Stress," by Miles O'Brien, Correspondent, and Jon Baime, Producer, *Science Nation*, National Science Foundation (www.nsf.gov), June 2011.

Results Of The Study

Both adults and teens reported feeling more afraid of the threat stimulus than the safety stimulus. Compared to adults, teens were less able to differentiate the threat from the safety stimulus.

Using functional magnetic resonance imaging, the researchers found that teens also had more activity in the hippocampus and right side of the amygdala than adults when viewing the threat stimulus compared with the safety stimulus. The hippocampus helps create and file new memories, while the amygdala activates the "fight-or-flight" response to stress and may be involved in fear learning.

Activity in another brain structure, the late-maturing dorsolateral prefrontal cortex (DLPFC), also differed between adults and teens. The DLPFC is highly involved in categorizing objects into different groups. In adults, activity increased as they rated more fear in relation to the safety stimulus. The researchers noted that this finding suggests that the adults' brains recruited the DLPFC more when they were unsure if a stimulus was safe or not safe. This uncertainty was reflected in their fear ratings.

Significance

The findings suggest that teen brains rely primarily on the hippocampus and right amygdala, brain structures that mature earlier in development and which are responsible for basic fear responses. In contrast, adults show more focused brain activity in prefrontal regions, which mature later in development. These regions are also involved in making more reasoned judgments about what is actually dangerous from what is safe.

According to the researchers, this difference may help to explain why teens generally report more pervasive worries and are more vulnerable to stress-related problems.

Chapter 4

Fight Or Flight Vs. Tend And Befriend

A New Stress Paradigm For Women

Rather than fighting or fleeing, women may respond to stress by tending to themselves and their young and befriending others.

Move over "fight-or-flight"—there's a new paradigm in town, the first new model to describe people's stress response patterns in more than 60 years.

The model, called "tend-and-befriend" by its developers, won't replace fight-or-flight. Rather, it adds another dimension to the stress-response arsenal, says University of California, Los Angeles, psychologist Shelley Taylor, PhD, who, along with five colleagues, developed the model.

In particular, they propose that females respond to stressful situations by protecting themselves and their young through nurturing behaviors—the "tend" part of the model—and forming alliances with a larger social group, particularly among women—the "befriend" part of the model. Males, in contrast, show less of a tendency toward tending and befriending, sticking more to the fight-or-flight response, they suggest.

The researchers describe this new model in an upcoming issue of *Psychological Review*, supporting their premise by pulling together existing evidence from research with nonhuman animals, neuroendocrine studies, and human-based social psychology.

The tend-and-befriend model fills what Taylor sees as a huge gap in the stress response literature: namely, that almost all the studies have been conducted in males and so, therefore, upheld fight-or-flight as the main response to stress.

The tend-and-befriend response, in contrast, fits better the way females respond to stress. It builds on the brain's attachment/caregiving system, which counteracts the metabolic activity associated with the traditional fight-or-flight stress response—increased heart rate, blood pressure, and cortisol levels—and leads to nurturing and affiliative behavior.

The research findings used to support the model are not new, says University of Chicago psychologist John Cacioppo, PhD, but the way they've been integrated is.

"The data supporting the model look very compelling," says Cacioppo, who has studied the biology of stress in animals and humans. "Even if it's wrong, which I don't think it will be, it's a very powerful model."

What's more, the model is sure to inspire thousands of new studies designed to test its claims, from whether women truly do respond to stress by tending and befriending, to questions about the specific hormonal and neuroendocrine systems responsible for the response to the specific contexts in which such a system may be triggered, adds psychologist Nancy Collins, PhD, who studies human reactions to stressful situations. The model can serve as a foundation on which to build an entirely new body of research, she says.

Culling The Evidence

Taylor and her colleagues developed their model after listening to a lecture on stress responses in rats. The description of fight-or-flight in response to stress didn't fit any of the findings Taylor had seen in almost 30 years as a health psychologist studying people's reactions to stressful life events.

When she began discussing the issue with her laboratory staff, postdoc Laura Klein, PhD, pointed out that the findings heard about at the lecture had been heavily based on studies of male animals.

"It was like a big light went on," says Taylor, who developed the new model with Klein, now at Pennsylvania State University; Brian Lewis, PhD, now at Syracuse University; Regan Gurung, PhD, now at the University of Wisconsin, Green Bay; and graduate students Tara Gruenewald and John Updegraff.

Women, they speculated, may have developed a completely different system for coping with stress in large part because their responses evolved in the context of being the primary caregiver of their children. To find support for their theory, they pulled together data from previously unconnected sources.

From research into the neuroendocrine responses responsible for fight-or-flight, for example, they document that, although women do show the same immediate hormonal and sympathetic nervous system response to acute stress, other factors intervene to make fight-or-flight less likely in females.

In terms of the fight response, while male aggression appears to be regulated by androgen hormones, such as testosterone, and linked to sympathetic reactivity and hostility, female aggression isn't. Instead, female aggression appears to be more cerebral in nature—moderated by social circumstances, learning, culture, and the situation—and in animals "confined to situations requiring defense," write the researchers.

In terms of flight, fleeing too readily at any sign of danger would put a female's offspring at risk, a response that might reduce her reproductive success in evolutionary terms. Consistent with this idea, studies in rats suggest there may be a physiological response to stress that inhibits flight. This response is the release of the hormone oxytocin, which enhances relaxation, reduces fearfulness and decreases the stress responses typical to the fight-or-flight response.

So rather than fight or flee, Taylor and her colleagues posit, women often tend and befriend, an idea supported by several lines of research in humans and other animals. Some of the more intriguing work, says Taylor, comes out of Michael Meaney's laboratory at McGill University. He and his colleagues remove rat pups from their nest for brief periods—a stressful situation for pups and mothers—and then return them to the nest and watch what happens. The mothers immediately move to nurture and soothe their pups by licking, grooming, and nursing them. This kind of tending response stimulates the growth of the pups' stress-regulatory system.

What stimulates this behavior in the mother? Taylor and her colleagues suggest that it's governed in part by oxytocin. Studies in many different animals, including non-human primates and humans, show that oxytocin promotes caregiving behavior and underlies attachment between mothers and their infants. In addition, some studies have found that mothers tend to be more nurturing and caring toward their children when they are most stressed.

As for the idea of "befriending" when stressed, Taylor and her colleagues detail evidence from rodent studies and studies in humans that when they are stressed, females prefer being with others, especially other females, while males don't. Indeed, in humans, women are much more likely than men to seek out and use social support in all types of stressful situations, including over health-related concerns, relationship problems, and work-related conflicts.

"It is one of the most robust gender differences in adult human behavior," write Taylor and her colleagues.

Again, oxytocin may be at play, they suggest. In female prairie voles, for example, injections of oxytocin enhance social contact and inhibit aggression. The same may occur in males, but males are less likely than females to have naturally high levels of oxytocin.

One Of A Repertoire Of Responses

Although the tend-and-befriend model emphasizes gender differences, the researchers reject the idea that gender stereotypes are written in our genes. Indeed, Taylor doesn't see biological models of behavior as inherently constraining—rather, they help tie human behavior to other species and provide a framework for general behavioral tendencies. The fun, she says, will be teasing apart how our biological predispositions unfold in the context of real-life experience.

Both Collins and Cacioppo hope that means researchers will examine social context to figure out which situations may promote tend-and-befriend and which might, instead, promote fight-or-flight or even as yet undiscovered stress responses.

Someone To Complain With Isn't Necessarily A Good Thing, Especially For Teenage Girls

New research shows that extensive discussion of problems may have a negative effect on emotional adjustment in girls.

Friendships that lend themselves to ruminating about problems may actually contribute to emotional difficulties in girls, according to new research. A study in the July issue of the journal *Developmental Psychology*, published by the American Psychological Association, finds that girls are more likely than boys of the same age group to develop anxiety and depression as a result of extensive conversations with friends about their problems.

Co-rumination, or excessively talking with another person about problems, including rehashing them and dwelling on the negative feelings associated with them, is thought to have both costs and benefits for people experiencing unpleasant situations. This six-month longitudinal study involved 813 third-, fifth-, seventh-, and ninth-grade girls and boys, and tested whether co-rumination is associated with depression and anxiety while simultaneously benefiting girls and boys by strengthening friendships.

For girls, co-rumination predicted increased positive friendship quality, including feelings of closeness between friends. However, the study also found that girls who co-ruminate had increased depressive and anxiety symptoms, which in turn, contributed to greater co-rumination.

"Having anxiety symptoms (and presumably, associated heightened levels of worries and concerns) and a high-quality friend to talk to may provide a uniquely reinforcing context for co-rumination," stated Amanda J. Rose, PhD, lead author and Associate Professor of Psychology at the University of Missouri—Columbia.

In fact, tend-and-befriend may be just as adaptive for men as for women in certain contexts, says Collins, whose research finds no gender differences when examining how often husbands and wives seek support from their most intimate companions—for example, each other.

"Perhaps these gender differences are adaptive with acute stressors," says Collins. "But when you think of longer term stressors, such as hunger, it doesn't make sense to have these gender differences. Men and women need social networks to work it out."

The most adaptive system would be one in which men and women select from a repertoire of responses depending on the specific stressor, she says.

Adds Taylor: Mainstream stress researchers "have been very quick to study behaviors like aggression and withdrawal and have failed to notice very important behaviors like affiliation. We think it's cute when women call up their sisters when they're under stress. But no one has realized that that is a contemporaneous manifestation of one of the oldest biological systems. Our focus on fight-or-flight has kept us from recognizing that there are systems that are as old as fight-or-flight that are tremendously important."

Rose and her colleagues speculated that co-rumination may lead girls to think about problems in a way that is different from boys, and that is more closely linked to emotional problems. For example, girls may be more likely than boys to take personal responsibility for failures, according to the study's authors.

For boys, co-rumination predicted only greater positive friendship quality and not increased depression and anxiety. "These findings are interesting because girls' intentions when discussing problems may be to give and seek positive support. However, these conversations appear to contribute to increased depression," said Rose.

The research cautions parents and adults against being lulled into a false sense of security about youth, especially girls, with seemingly supportive friendships. While other studies indicate that adults should worry about socially isolated youth, this research raises the issue that youth in seemingly supportive friendships may also be at risk for depression and anxiety if the friendship is based on a pattern of co-rumination.

For more information: Read "Prospective Associations of Co-Rumination with Friendship and Emotional Adjustment Considering the Socioemotional Trade-Offs of Co-Rumination" at http://www.apa.org/pubs/journals/releases/dev-4341019.pdf.

Part Two
Common Causes Of Stress In Teens

Chapter 5

What Causes Stress In Kids?

The Kids Aren't All Right

There's a disconnect between what children say they're worrying about and what their parents think is stressing them, a gap that could have long-term implications for children's mental and physical health, according to the American Psychological Association's (APA's) latest "Stress in America" research.

Children age 8–17 say they worry about doing well in school, getting into good colleges, and their family's finances. They also report suffering headaches, sleeplessness, and upset stomachs.

But these stresses and symptoms are going largely unnoticed by parents, survey findings show.

In fact, more than one in three children report experiencing headaches in the past month, but only 13 percent of parents think their children experience headaches as a result of stress. In addition, while 44 percent of children report sleeping difficulties, only 13 percent of parents think their kids have trouble sleeping.

The survey also found that about one-fifth of children reported they worry a great deal or a lot, but only three percent of parents rate their children's stress as extreme (an eight, nine, or 10 on a 10-point scale). In addition, almost 30 percent of children worried about their families' financial difficulties, but just 18 percent of parents thought that was a source of worry for their children.

The findings are troubling because chronic stress left untreated can contribute to psychological problems as well as physical conditions, says Katherine Nordal, PhD, APA's executive director for professional practice. She says parents need to make themselves available and let their children know it's OK to approach them if they're worried about something.

"Parents need to be intentional about setting aside time to be available to their children," she says. "If parents aren't receptive, kids may feel like they're being an additional burden on their parents by talking about their problems."

The online survey, conducted by Harris Interactive for the third consecutive year for the Practice Directorate's ongoing Mind/Body Health public education campaign, polled a nationally representative sample of 1,568 adults in July and August. Results for children age 8–17 were drawn from a YouthQuery survey of 1,206 young people conducted online by Harris in August.

Women Still More Stressed

The findings for adults are also troubling:

- Stress levels are high, with 42 percent of adults indicating their stress worsened in the past year. A total of 24 percent said they had an extreme level of stress (eight, nine, or 10 on a 10-point scale) over the past month, and 51 percent report moderate stress levels (four to seven on a 10-point scale).

- About two-thirds of respondents said they've been diagnosed by a physician with a chronic condition, most commonly high blood pressure or high cholesterol. Seventy percent said a health-care provider recommended lifestyle or behavior changes. That data also show that adults who were advised to make lifestyle changes may not have received enough support from their physicians to do so. In fact, fewer than half were told by their physicians why the changes were important; only 35 percent were given tips or shown techniques for making changes; and only five percent to 10 percent were referred to another health-care provider for follow-up. Similar to last year's results, women report having experienced more stress symptoms than men, such as irritability or anger, fatigue and depression.

- Among parents of 8- to 17-year-olds, mothers reported higher levels of stress than fathers. On a scale of one to 10 (with 10 being the highest level), 15 percent of moms rated their stress as a 10, compared with only three percent of dads. Mothers were also more likely to report lying awake at night, eating unhealthy foods, overeating or skipping a meal because of stress.

Such findings underscore the need for psychologists to work within the nation's health-care system to help people make needed lifestyle and behavioral changes, Nordal says.

"The key in managing stress effectively for both physical and mental well-being is having effective coping strategies, a combination of relaxation strategies along with exercise, combined with good sleep habits and good eating habits," she says.

This is particularly important for women who often face a "second shift" of caring for children and running a household when they get home from work, says Helen Coons, PhD, a Philadelphia-based clinical health psychologist who works primarily with women. "The reality is, so many women are just too tired. They're running on empty."

That calls for change at several levels to support women, says Coons. Workplaces should offer better access to day care and more flexibility to allow women time for medical checkups and exercise breaks. Spouses or partners need to watch the kids while mom goes out for a run or a brisk walk, and neighborhood families can rotate babysitting to give parents more flexibility.

"There's that African saying, it takes a village to raise a child. I think it takes a community to support women and families" for healthier lifestyles, she says.

Mile-High Stress

This year's survey also took snapshots of how Americans are faring with stress in eight metropolitan areas—Atlanta, Chicago, Denver, Detroit, Los Angeles, New York, Seattle, and Washington, DC—comparing results with national findings.

Fairing the worst was Denver, where more than 75 percent of residents report that work and money are significant sources of stress, and 35 percent rated their stress as extreme over the prior month.

That distress sounds familiar to Stephanie Smith, PsyD, public education coordinator for the Colorado Psychological Association and a Denver-based practitioner. Although the city's unemployment rate isn't as high as the national average, many of her clients tell her they feel trapped at their jobs. They're working harder for less money because of layoffs and pay cuts, but they're unable to find better jobs and frightened of losing their health insurance.

Smith works with her clients to identify things they can do to relieve stress, such as spending more quality time with family and exercising. "We talk about the things you can control in your life," she says.

In Los Angeles, 71 percent of respondents said they've been told by a health provider they have a chronic condition, compared with 66 percent nationally.

Table 5.1. What Stresses Teens Out?

Becky Beacom, health education manager for Palo Alto Medical Foundation (PAMF), surveyed 124 adolescents to explore what they find most stressful. Find out what gives your peers stress below.

Issue	Number Of Times Mentioned	Percent
Homework/School	138	55%
• Grades/GPA		
• Tests		
• College		
• Finals week		
Parents/Family	37	15%
• Expectations		
• Pressure to do well		
• Not achieving/ blowing it		
Social Life	22	(9%)
• Friends		
• Boyfriends/Girlfriends		
• Relationships		
• Extracurriculars		
• Try outs		
• Shows		
• Sex		
Time	20	8%
• No time		
• Deadlines		
• Keeping up		
• Lack of sleep		
• Doing two things at once		
• Too much going on		
• Unprepared		
Sports	**10**	4%
Other	22	9%

Source: "What Stresses Teens Out?" reprinted with permission from the Palo Alto Medical Foundation Teen Health website, http://www.pamf.org/teen, © 2012 Palo Alto Medical Foundation. All rights reserved.

Table 5.2. Sources Of Stress By Age

Questions asked parents appear in *italics*; questions asked [youth] appear in **bold**.

	Parents			**Youth**		
	Total	8–12	13–17	Total	8–12	13–17
	N=235	101	134	1,206	536	670
*Managing school pressures/responsibilities/ homework/grades/***Doing well in school**	34%	31%	36%	44%	44%	43%
*Relationships with siblings/***Getting along with my brother(s) or sister(s)**	17%	17%	16%	8%	14%	2%
*Relationships with peers/***Getting along with my friends**	20%	20%	20%	16%	22%	11%
*Your family's financial difficulties/***My family having enough money**	18%	20%	17%	30%	28%	31%
*His/her physical appearance/weight/***The way I look/My weight**	17%	17%	17%	22%	17%	26%
*Your relationship with your spouse/partner/***My parent(s)/guardian or other family members arguing or fighting more**	12%	16%	9%	10%	14%	7%
*Pressure managing extracurricular commitments (e.g., sports, hobbies)/***Managing activities such as sports, music, clubs, etc.**	12%	12%	12%	10%	7%	12%
*Peer pressure to engage in risky behaviors (e.g., smoking, drinking, drugs, sex, etc.)/***Pressure from friends who want me to try smoking, drinking, drugs, sex, etc.**	6%	1%	10%	2%	–	3%
*Getting into a good college/Determining future/***Getting into a good college/Deciding what to do after high school**	3%	1%	5%	17%	5%	29%
Non-financial pressures on family members (e.g., health, job frustrations, getting along with extended family, etc.)	3%	3%	4%	N/A	N/A	N/A
Getting along with my boyfriend or girlfriend	N/A	N/A	N/A	3%	1%	4%
My parents(s)/guardian losing their jobs	N/A	N/A	N/A	6%	7%	6%
Other [Asked of parents and youth]	8%	10%	6%	10%	12%	8%

"To me, that's absolutely frightening, because we know the role stress plays in wearing our bodies down," says Michael Ritz, PhD, co-chair of the California Psychological Association's public education steering committee.

Psychologists can help people manage their stress and live healthier lifestyles, Ritz says.

"That underscores so much why psychologists need to be part of our health-care team," he says.

Chapter 6

Teens And Stress: Are You Overbooked?

- "How much stress is normal? It's hard for me to go even a day without stressing about everything from writing a paper to making the soccer team."

- "I couldn't handle all my honors classes last year, but I know colleges love AP credits and my parents want me to go to a good school. How can I explain that I can't do it all anymore?"

- "I'm like a juggler who's afraid to drop one of the million balls I've got up in the air. I can't relax without feeling like everything will come crashing down on me."

Do you recognize these feelings of being stressed and overbooked? What conscientious teen hasn't felt overwhelmed by expectations at some point or another? It's important to know that there are different types of stress and not all stress is bad. Having some degree of stress in your life can be motivating; it may push you to achieve things you never before thought you were capable of accomplishing. When you find yourself saddled with too much stress, however, you may be tempted to give up on everything, even those activities and challenges you enjoy.

According to Benjamin Hunnicutt, professor of leisure studies at the University of Iowa, "Overbooked kids are a real danger in a society where work is taking on more and more importance in adults' lives." Children watch their parents go about their daily schedules, and they can't help but notice when work starts to sap the time that used to go to family and community activities. "We're living in a time when adults' lives have become more scheduled

About This Chapter: "Teens And Stress: Are You Overbooked?" *Decisions,* Winter 2005 newsletter. Reprinted with permission from SADD, Inc. (http://sadd.org), © 2005. Reviewed by Dr. David A. Cooke, MD, FACP, March 2013.

and more hectic, and children seem to be encouraged to join the pace at an earlier age than ever before," says Hunnicutt. No wonder many teens are feeling burned out by the time they reach high school!

It's certainly important to find activities you enjoy and to commit to them. Whether it's a part-time job after school, community service through your church, or playing varsity sports, learning to be a responsible member of a group is part of growing up and can be a lot of fun. When you find that your schedule has crossed the line from rewarding to completely overwhelming, however, you may find you are doing yourself more harm than good.

Often the difference between successful and unsuccessful people is their ability to manage time. There is no magic formula to knowing just how many activities are appropriate; that depends on how you deal with the pressures and commitment each one requires. If you're a person who values free time above other endeavors, you need to remember this when you're choosing your commitments. Perhaps adding another night of drama practice won't bring you as much enjoyment as having a free night to chill out on your own. On the other hand, if you're a person who thrives in structured scheduling, you might be able to handle joining the choir when you're already treasurer of Students Against Destructive Decisions (SADD) and captain of the swimming team. The secret to being happy, healthy, and successful during these important years is finding your own way to balance the things you need to do with the things you enjoy doing.

Parents need to take responsibility too. Millions of children and teens across the country feel overwhelmed and pressured. Psychologist Alvin Rosenfield, MD, author of *The Over-Scheduled Child: Avoiding the Hyper-Parenting Trap*, believes that enrolling kids in too many activities is a trend that has spread nationwide. "Overscheduling our children is not only a widespread phenomenon, it's also how we parent today," he says. "Parents think that they're not being good parents if their kids aren't in all kinds of activities. Children are under pressure to achieve, to be competitive. I know sixth-graders who are already working on their resumes so they'll have an edge when they apply to college." In fact, colleges do not want students who "dabble" in many activities. They want students who are committed to school and to those activities that they do best.

Other experts echo Rosenfield's observations. "Kids in America are so overscheduled that they have no [free] time. They have no time to call on their own resources and be creative. Creativity is making something out of nothing, and it takes time for that to happen," says Diane Ehrensaft, PhD, of the Wright Institute. "In our efforts to raise Renaissance children who are competitive in all areas, we squelch creativity." This type of pressure can leave kids feeling overwhelmed and stressed out.

Signs You Are Stressed

Worried about work, money, friends, or family? Sometimes stress can build up before you know it and leave you feeling overwhelmed. Take a look at these signs of stress and find out how to recognize stress before it takes over.

You know you're stressed if:

1. You eat standing up.
2. Your dog doesn't recognize you.
3. You're always late.
4. You forget what day it is.
5. You have trouble finishing a sentence.
6. Your friends greet you, "Hey, stranger!"
7. You're drinking more than usual.
8. You're fighting more than usual.
9. You can't remember what "usual" is.
10. You do three things at once; you don't finish any of them.
11. You lose your keys. And your glasses. And your patience.
12. You only talk to people via e-mail.
13. You're always tired.
14. You can't sleep.
15. You keep getting sick.
16. You keep dropping things.
17. You bite your nails, tap your feet, and twirl your hair. All at the same time.
18. You feel like you're drowning.
19. You don't have time to feed your fish.
20. Your blood pressure is too high.
21. Your morale is too low.
22. You jump when the phone rings.
23. You eat. And eat. And eat.
24. You have a headache. Again.
25. Your palms are sweaty.
26. Your heart is racing.
27. You feel nervous or jumpy.
28. Nothing seems fun anymore.
29. You snap at your friends.
30. Your socks don't match.
31. You yell at your partner.
32. You hate getting up in the morning.
33. You drive too fast.
34. You talk too fast.
35. You cry at the drop of a hat.
36. You can't breathe.
37. You can't concentrate.
38. You keep bumping into things.
39. You can't see over the laundry.
40. You're never alone.
41. You're always alone.
42. You live on coffee, cigarettes, or diet soda.
43. You haven't opened the mail in days.
44. It's always someone else's fault.
45. People keep asking: "Are you okay?"
46. You wonder if you are okay.

A pioneer in the field of stress research, Hans Slye, MD, describes two different types of stress that teens feel: eustress and distress. Eustress is the pleasant stress we feel when we confront the normal challenges of life. A teen who loves basketball may thrive on the pressures of practices and games. Distress, on the other hand, occurs when we feel overwhelmed. The same kid who loves basketball may start to see it as a burden when it becomes one of four or five other activities.

The key to solving this problem seems to lie in one word: balance. Finding the happy medium between scheduled activities and free time will keep most teens on an even keel. If you find yourself overbooked, take a serious look at where your time is going. Prioritize things that you must do (i.e., going to school) and then find some time for the one or two things you most want to do. If hockey is fun but it takes time away from your real passion, playing drums in a band, it might be time to hang up your skates.

Enjoying a few activities and doing them well will always bring you more satisfaction than stretching yourself too thin by trying to do everything.

Chapter 7

Current Events And Stress: News You Can Use

The news can be full of stories about unexpected or bad things like tornadoes or hurricanes, disease threats, bombings, kidnappings, and war. And the scary thing is—it may seem like these things are happening all around you, even in places where you feel secure like school, the mall, and at home. Seeing these things on TV or even experiencing them first hand (like being in a tornado) can cause you to feel uncertain, worried, or scared. These feelings may last even after the event is over.

Here are some tips to understanding the news and what you see and hear:

- **The news doesn't talk about everyday activities.** Instead, the news talks about things that are out of the ordinary—both good and bad. And sometimes it seems like the news shows more of the bad stuff—things like tragedies and crime. For example, if a plane crashes, it will get a lot of attention in the news—so much so, that you may think planes crash all the time. But in fact, thousands of planes take off and land safely each day—the news just doesn't talk about it.

- **Sometimes you see stories over and over again.** The news may talk about tragic events (like bombings) or disasters (such as floods, earthquakes, or hurricanes) repeatedly, but this doesn't mean these things are happening all the time—it just means that the news is talking about it again. The news will cover something when it first happens and then repeat the story. So you may see it on the news when you get home from school and then again before you go to bed. After the first day, the news may do what is called a "follow-up" story to tell you what happened after the event, so you may hear about the same thing for a few days, even though it only happened once.

About This Chapter: Information for this chapter is excerpted from "News You Can Use," BAM! Body And Mind, Centers for Disease Control and Prevention (www.bam.gov). January 2013.

- **Bad things in the news can alert you.** For example, a news story could tell you about someone in your community who is breaking into homes. While this may scare you, just remember that even though it's on the news, that doesn't mean it will happen to you. But stories like this can help make you aware of your surroundings and of things you can do to protect yourself (like locking your doors).

- **Disasters or tragic events can bring out the best in people.** Firemen and policemen are doing their jobs (like saving people), and volunteers and everyday citizens may also be there to help. You will see people in your community volunteering to bring food and clothing to help people who are affected, families coming together to help each other out, and shelters being put into place to give people a place to stay.

- **It is normal to be concerned**. It is important to know, though, that while things may seem uncertain for a while, your life usually will return to normal fairly soon.

Weave Your Own Safety Net

Following these tips can help you get on with your day-to-day life, even during stressful times.

- **Talk to your friends and your family and spend time with them.** If you find yourself feeling unsafe, uncertain, worried, or scared, or if you don't understand what is going on around you, talk to your parents, teachers, or a school counselor. Your parents or other adults can help explain these events so you can understand things better. By talking with your friends and your family, you can share your feelings and know you are not alone. Plus, spending time with them may help you feel more safe and secure.

- **Help out others.** Sometimes when you are concerned about what is going on around you, it is helpful to give others support. You can help out by raising money, donating clothes, or organizing an event like a food drive at your school to collect food and/or supplies for an organization that helps people affected by war, terrorism, or natural disasters. Even if you and your family are the ones who are affected by a disaster, helping others can help you deal with your own stress—it may make you feel a little more in control.

- **Write your feelings down.** Writing your feelings down in a diary, a journal, or even on a piece of scrap paper is a great way to get things off of your chest. You can write down how you feel, what's going on in your life, or anything else.

- **Stick to your normal routine.** There is comfort in the little things you do every day—so keep on doing them. And take care of yourself. Get lots of sleep, eat well, and be physically active.

- **Take a break from the news.** Watch a funny movie, play some games, go outside and play, or read a funny book or magazine. Too much information about disasters can get you down, so change your pace and watch some cartoons, read a joke book, or even make up your own. Did you know that smiling has been proven to improve your mood? That can help you feel like new and take your mind off things for a while.

Plan Ahead

Sometimes things happen that we just can't anticipate, but a few things (like hurricanes, tornadoes, or forest fires) occur in certain areas of the country during certain seasons. If you live in areas where weather "can take you by storm," you can take a few steps to help prepare in case of an emergency. Being prepared can help you feel like you have more control in an emergency, and help you feel less stressed.

- **Make a plan.** Talk to your parents about being prepared. Just like your family should have a plan to get out of the house in case of a fire, make a plan in case bad weather strikes. Choose a place to go, who you would call, or what you would do. Make sure to talk about what you should do if you are at school, or a friend's house, or if your parents are at work.

- **Have an emergency supply kit.** During or after a storm, you may be without power for a few days or you may not be able to leave your home. Work with your parents to put together a supply kit for such emergencies. Some things to have on hand include water, and non-perishable (that means they won't spoil) foods such as crackers, peanut butter, and canned food (soup, fruit, veggies, etc.). Make sure to have a battery-powered radio, flashlights, and extra batteries on hand. A first-aid kit, facial tissue, and toilet paper are good things to consider packing. Lanterns (lamp oil) or candles for light are good things to have too. Also, don't forget about your family pet. Pack extra water and food for your four-legged friends.

- **Put together an activity survival kit.** Having some favorite books and games on hand will keep you interested and help pass the time. While you may not want to live without power forever, being without it for a few days may be fun—it could give you an idea of what life was like before electricity.

Chapter 8

What Stresses You Out About School?

A new school year is exciting. There's that wonderful feeling of making a fresh start, catching up with old friends, and making progress by moving up a grade. But there's no denying that it can be stressful too.

What's Worrying You

If you find yourself preparing for school by hoping for the best and imagining the worst, you're not alone. Here's what we heard from 600 people who took our survey on back-to-school worries.

One third said they worry most about schoolwork. No surprise there. You'll be studying more advanced material, so it's natural to worry about whether you'll do OK.

But not everyone said schoolwork was their biggest worry. Just as many people said they worry most about social issues like fitting in, having friends, being judged, or being teased. Since social life is such a big part of school, it's not a shock that social issues are the biggest worry for some people.

Besides schoolwork and social stuff, another category ranked high on the worry list: appearance. One-fourth of the people who responded to our survey said appearance issues worried them most of all. If this is you, you've got plenty of company.

About This Chapter: "What Stresses You Out About School" is reprinted with permission from www.kidshealth .org. This information was provided by KidsHealth®, one of the largest resources online for medically reviewed health information written for parents, kids, and teens. For more articles like this, visit www.KidsHealth.org or www.TeensHealth.org. Copyright © 1995–2012 The Nemours Foundation. All rights reserved.

Kimberly, 14, told us, "I'm happy about going back to school—I'm bored stiff here! But I'm worried about reputation, teasing, failing, and being a nerd."

So we asked people to tell us how they plan to cope with the things that worry them most, and whether they have advice for others. You can see what they said on the following pages.

What Worries You Most About Going Back To School?

Schoolwork issues: 32%

Social issues: 30%

Appearance issues: 25%

Nothing: 10%

Extracurricular issues: 3%

Managing Worries About Schoolwork

Rachel, 15, told us, "I'm kind [of] hard on myself, like I feel really bad if I don't have a 4.0 grade average."

Lots of people are hard on themselves, but worrying can just add to the pressure. Casey, 15, offered this advice: "Stressing too much about it doesn't get you anywhere. It's good to be concerned about your work, but you have to act on that."

Here are some of the plans you have for coping with schoolwork:

- Zach, 18, said, "Better time management. I need to stop talking with the social butterflies and get to work!"

- Michael, 16, plans to "come home, take a quick break, and then get started on my work straight away. Procrastination only brings frustration!"

- Katie, 17, offered this advice: "To avoid trouble, do [your] homework as soon as possible and at least start projects the day you get them."

Finding The Right Balance—And Support

Fallon, 16, said, "Finding time for everything is going to be a challenge!"

Daniel, 14, agreed. "I play sports so I have to keep my grades up to play." How does he keep the balance? "Work really hard and lean on my parents for lots of support. If you have parents around that actually take an interest in you, take advantage of that and let them be there for you."

Relying on other people for support and advice can help balance all the pressures school can bring. [Here are some ideas for finding the right balance:]

- Claire, 15, depends on her brother. "He is 18 and has been through it."

- Dana, 14, advised, "Use the guidance counselor. That's why they are there."

- Chelsea, 16, said her teachers were a big help when she was trying to catch up in school: "Since I asked for help I've felt more relaxed and more normal so that now it doesn't bother me as much as it did."

Balancing school with life's other demands means staying healthy. Lots of people told us their goal for the school year is to eat well, get plenty of exercise, and lots of sleep so they'll be primed to succeed.

Managing Social Pressures And Problems

When it comes to the social scene, making new friends is one of the biggest worries people mentioned. Lots of people said that friends would be in different classes or even at different schools.

Jessie, 15, said, "I'm going to try to make new friends and talk more. Don't worry about being awkward because others are too. Lots of people are good at being cool, but they are insecure too."

Finding a safe, welcoming group is a great foundation for dealing with the ups and downs of school. Jessie's advice: "It's important to have your own little or big group that you can hang out with."

Lolo, 14, explained how "My best friend left last year, and I'm worried about who I'll hang out with." Her strategy is: "Don't hang out with anyone who has a good social image but who is mean. Try to find someone who will really be your friend."

Lots of people are concerned about drifting apart from friends and breaking away from existing friendships to start new ones.

Jen, 16, told us, "I have not talked to my best friends all summer. I don't want to be their friend anymore, but they don't get that."

Leanna, 14, said, "I am stressed about the groups and who I am going to sit with because I have different friends in different groups."

Tim, 14, worried about "making new friends without ex-friends spreading rumors."

Brittany, 15, who worried about dealing with "rude old friends," offered this advice: "Be nice to everyone. You never know who you may need help from in the future."

And Amina, 14, said, "There are these really jealous girls and they are always stressing me out." She found that just being nice to them can make a lot of difference: "They will be amazed at how you treat them and maybe loosen up some."

Using kindness to stop meanness in its tracks is one good way to deal. Jessica, 16, has another strategy for coping with rude people: "I just ignore them. It drives them crazy when you don't act or seem like you care about anything they have to say."

Some of you worry that the things you did in the past will influence how people see you now. Tina, 15, told us, "My best friend and I were in a car accident last year when we decided to go to a party instead of school. So I am worried that my peers and teachers will think that I am irresponsible because of that incident."

Amanda, 14, said her way of dealing with rumors and gossip is "to hold my head up high, smile, and try to create a new reputation for myself. Change the negatives into positives!"

Looking Good

How we feel about the way we look is closely tied to social issues, feeling comfortable, and being accepted.

Codi, 14, said, "I am not usually a shy person, but starting high school in a new school is scary. I don't know anyone other than those on my soccer team. I am afraid that once they see me out of my soccer clothes and in my skater cut-up clothes they won't want to talk to me."

"At my old school, I was the most popular girl," said Emily, 14. "Now I'm starting to get acne and developing." Dealing with body changes is a big issue for lots of people.

It's natural to worry about appearance, but most people said they try to keep things in perspective.

Casey, 14, said, "A year from now, will what you worried about really be a big deal? Other stuff is going to happen."

Lots of you recommend getting the support of a friend, parent, or counselor when you're feeling down about your appearance.

Keisha, 15, said, "Don't worry about it so much. And when your family and friends say you look great, accept the compliment, because it's true!"

Mickie, 14, told us she has no worries about starting school, but she does have this advice for looking good on the first day: "Wear clothes that fit your style. Don't wear something that makes you look like a poser."

And Lia, 14, reminds us, "If you're worried about your clothes and how you look, just remember that it's what's on the inside that matters."

We couldn't agree more.

Stress Relief Advice From Teens

- "When you are having a tough time, find something you like to do. For me, it's working at the animal shelter. It helps to take your mind off things." —Haley, 14
- "Try to find your ultimate soother. I found mine: music! Whenever things worry me, I put my headphones on and forget about my problems for a while. —Ashlee, 14
- "Do something that de-stresses you, like drawing or reading a book or listening to music or writing—or, of course, scream in your pillow." —Ann Marie, 14
- "I go out and run." —Shane, 14

Chapter 9

Test Anxiety

You've participated in class, done all of your homework, studied hard, and you think you have a grip on the material. But then the day of the test comes. Suddenly, you blank out, freeze up, zone out, or feel so nervous that you can't get it together to respond to those questions you knew the answers to just last night.

If this sounds like you, you may have a case of test anxiety—that nervous feeling that people sometimes get when they're about to take a test.

It's pretty normal to feel a little nervous and stressed before a test. Just about everyone does. And a touch of nervous anticipation can actually help you get revved and keep you at peak performance while you're taking the test. But for some people, this normal anxiety is more intense. The nervousness they feel before a test can be so strong that it interferes with their concentration or performance.

What is test anxiety?

Test anxiety is actually a type of *performance anxiety*—a feeling someone might have in a situation where performance really counts or when the pressure's on to do well. For example, a person might experience performance anxiety when he or she is about to try out for the school play, sing a solo on stage, get into position at the pitcher's mound, step onto the platform in a diving meet, or go into an important interview.

About This Chapter: Information in this chapter is from "Test Anxiety," July 2010, reprinted with permission from www.kidshealth.org. This information was provided by KidsHealth®, one of the largest resources online for medically reviewed health information written for parents, kids, and teens. For more articles like this, visit www .KidsHealth.org or www.TeensHealth.org. Copyright © 1995–2012 The Nemours Foundation. All rights reserved.

Like other situations in which a person might feel performance anxiety, test anxiety can bring on "butterflies," a stomachache, or a tension headache. Some people might feel shaky, sweaty, or feel their heart beating quickly as they wait for the test to be given out. A student with really strong test anxiety may even feel like he or she might pass out or throw up.

Test anxiety is not the same as doing poorly on a certain test because your mind is on something else. Most people know that having other things on their minds—such as a breakup or the death of someone close—can also interfere with their concentration and prevent them from doing their best on a test.

What causes it?

All anxiety is a reaction to anticipating something stressful. Like other anxiety reactions, test anxiety affects the body and the mind. When you're under stress, your body releases the hormone adrenaline, which prepares it for danger (you may hear this referred to as the "fight or flight" reaction). That's what causes the physical symptoms, such as sweating, a pounding heart, and rapid breathing. These sensations might be mild or intense.

Focusing on the bad things that could happen also fuels test anxiety. For example, someone worrying about doing poorly might think thoughts like, "What if I forget everything I know?" or "What if the test is too hard?" Too many thoughts like these leave no mental space for thinking about the test questions. People with test anxiety can also feel stressed out by their physical reaction and think things like "What if I throw up?" or "Oh no, my hands are shaking."

Just like other types of anxiety, test anxiety can create a vicious circle: The more a person focuses on the bad things that could happen, the stronger the feeling of anxiety becomes. This makes the person feel worse and, because his or her head is full of distracting thoughts and fears, it can increase the possibility that the person will do worse on the test.

Who's likely to have test anxiety?

People who worry a lot or who are perfectionists are more likely to have trouble with test anxiety. People with these traits sometimes find it hard to accept mistakes they might make or to get anything less than a perfect score. In this way, even without meaning to, they might really pressure themselves. Test anxiety is bound to thrive in a situation like this.

Students who aren't prepared for tests but who care about doing well are also likely to experience test anxiety. If you know you're not prepared, it's a no-brainer to realize that you'll be worried about doing poorly. People can feel unprepared for tests for several reasons: They may not have studied enough, they may find the material difficult, or perhaps they feel tired because didn't get enough sleep the night before.

What can you do?

Test anxiety can be a real problem if you're so stressed out over a test that you can't get past the nervousness to focus on the test questions and do your best work. Feeling ready to meet the challenge, though, can keep test anxiety at a manageable level.

Use a little stress to your advantage. Stress is your body's warning mechanism—it's a signal that helps you prepare for something important that's about to happen. So use it to your advantage. Instead of reacting to the stress by dreading, complaining, or fretting about the test with friends, take an active approach. Let stress remind you to study well in advance of a test. Chances are, you'll keep your stress from spinning out of control. After all, nobody ever feels stressed out by thoughts that they might do well on a test.

Ask for help. Although a little test anxiety can be a good thing, an overdose of it is another story entirely. If sitting for a test gets you so stressed out that your mind goes blank and causes you to miss answers that you know, then your level of test anxiety probably needs some attention. Your teacher, your school guidance counselor, or a tutor can be useful resources to talk to if you always get extreme test anxiety.

Be prepared. Some students think that going to class is all it should take to learn and do well on tests. But there's much more to learning than just hoping to soak everything up in class. That's why good study habits and skills are so important—and why no amount of cramming or studying the night before a test can take the place of the deeper level of learning that happens over time with regular study.

Many students find that their test anxiety is reduced when they start to study better or more regularly. It makes sense—the more you know the material, the more confident you'll feel. Having confidence going into a test means you expect to do well. When you expect to do well, you'll be able to relax into a test after the normal first-moment jitters pass.

Watch what you're thinking. If expecting to do well on a test can help you relax, what about when people expect they won't do well? Watch out for any negative messages you might be sending yourself about the test. They can contribute to your anxiety.

If you find yourself thinking negative thoughts ("I'm never any good at taking tests" or "It's going to be terrible if I do badly on this test"), replace them with positive messages. Not unrealistic positive messages, of course, but ones that are practical and true, such as "I've studied hard and I know the material, so I'm ready to do the best I can." (Of course, if you haven't studied, this message won't help!)

Accept mistakes. Another thing you can do is to learn to keep mistakes in perspective—especially if you're a perfectionist or you tend to be hard on yourself. Everyone makes mistakes, and you may have even heard teachers or coaches refer to mistakes as "learning opportunities." Learning to tolerate small failures and mistakes—like that one problem you got wrong in the math pop quiz—is a valuable skill.

Take care of yourself. It can help to learn ways to calm yourself down and get centered when you're tense or anxious. For some people, this might mean learning a simple breathing exercise. Practicing breathing exercises regularly (when you're not stressed out) helps your body see these exercises as a signal to relax.

And, of course, taking care of your health—such as getting enough sleep, exercise, and healthy eats before a test—can help keep your mind working at its best.

Everything takes time and practice, and learning to beat test anxiety is no different. Although it won't go away overnight, facing and dealing with test anxiety will help you learn stress management, which can prove to be a valuable skill in many situations besides taking tests.

Chapter 10

Peer Pressure

Your classmates keep asking you to have them over because you have a pool, everyone at school is wearing silly hats so you do too, and your best friend begs you to go running with her because you both need more exercise, so you go, too. These are all examples of peer pressure. Don't get it yet?

- **Pressure** is the feeling that you are being pushed toward making a certain choice—good or bad.

- **A peer** is someone in your own age group.

- **Peer pressure** is—you guessed it—the feeling that someone your own age is pushing you toward making a certain choice, good or bad.

What's so difficult about avoiding peer pressure? People want to be accepted and liked by people their own age.

Why Peer Pressure Can Work

Have you ever given in to pressure? Like when a friend begs to borrow something you don't want to give up or to do something your parents say is off limits? Chances are you probably have given into pressure at some time in your life.

How did it feel to give into pressure? If you did something you wish you hadn't, then most likely you didn't feel too good about it. You might have felt some of these feelings:

About This Chapter: Information in this chapter is excerpted from "Peer Pressure: Why Peer Pressure Can Work," The Cool Spot, U.S. Department of Health and Human Services (www.thecoolspot.gov), 2010.

- Sad
- Anxious
- Guilty
- Like a wimp or pushover
- Disappointed in yourself

How Peers Pressure

Almost everyone faces peer pressure once in a while. Friends have a big influence on our lives, but sometimes they push us to do things that we may not want to do. Unless you want to give in every time you face this, you're going to need to learn how to handle it.

The first step to standing up to peer pressure is to understand it. In this section, you'll start by learning to recognize the different things people do when they pressure others. Check out the differences between spoken and unspoken pressures, and learn about the peer pressure bag of tricks.

Soon you'll be able to spot peer pressure and deal with it!

Spoken Versus Unspoken Pressure

Sometimes a friend can say something directly to you that puts a lot of pressure on you and makes it hard to say no. This is **spoken** pressure.

Or, you may think you are supposed to act or dress a certain way because it seems like everyone else is doing it, or because it's the cool thing to do. When you feel this way even though nobody has said anything about it, this is **unspoken** pressure.

If you haven't already, you are going to face both spoken and unspoken pressure in the future. It's just part of life. The important part is to make the right choices when a peer pressure situation comes up.

Peer Pressure Bag Of Tricks

Who needs you as a friend anyway? You're such a baby! It won't hurt bad!

Have your friends ever used these lines on you? Did you give in, even though you didn't want to?

These are a few of the goodies in the Peer Pressure Bag-of-Tricks. The tricks include put-downs, rejections, and reasoning, as well as pressure without words, or unspoken pressure.

The Right To Resist

If someone is pressuring you to do anything that's not right or good for you, you have the right to resist. You have the right to say no, the right not to give a reason why, and the right to just walk away from a situation.

Resisting pressure can be hard for some people. Why? Here are a few reasons:

- They are afraid of being rejected by others.
- They want to be liked and don't want to lose a friend.
- They want to appear grown up.
- They don't want to be made fun of by others.
- They don't want to hurt someone's feelings.
- They aren't sure of what they really want.
- They don't know how to get out of the situation.

Sometimes resisting isn't easy, but you can do it with practice and a little know-how. Keep trying, even if you don't get it right at first.

To get started, check out these Quick Tips on resisting pressure:

- Say no and let them know you mean it.
- Stand up straight.
- Make eye contact.
- Say how you feel.
- Don't make excuses.
- Stick up for yourself.

The Tricks

Learn to spot the tricks. Being aware of the pressure is the first step to resisting it.

- **Rejection:** Threatening to end a friendship or a relationship. This pressure can be hard to resist because nobody wants to lose friends. Some examples of pressure by rejection are:

    - Who needs you as a friend anyway?

    - If you don't drink, we won't hang out any more.

    - Why don't you leave if you don't want to drink with us?

- **Put Downs:** Insulting or calling a person names to make them feel bad. Some examples of put downs are:

  - You're never any fun.

  - You're such a baby.

  - You're such a wimp.

  - You're so uncool.

- **Reasoning:** Telling a person reasons why they should try something or why it would be OK if they did. (Nobody said these were good reasons.) Some examples of pressure by reasoning are:

  - It won't hurt you.

  - Your parents will never find out.

  - You'll have more fun.

Unspoken Pressure

This is something you feel without anyone saying anything to you. You feel unspoken pressure if you want to do the same things others doing. Some unspoken pressure tricks are:

- **The Huddle:** A group of kids standing together in which everyone is talking and maybe looking at something you can't see, laughing, and joking.

- **The Look:** Kids who think they're cool give you a certain look that means we're cool and you're not.

- **The Example:** A group of popular kids decide to get the same backpack and you want one too.

Peer Pressure Can Be Good Too

Peer pressure isn't all bad. You and your friends can pressure each other into some things that will improve your health and social life and make you feel good about your decisions.

Think of a time when a friend pushed you to do something good for yourself or to avoid something that would've been bad. Here are some good things friends can pressure each other to do:

- Be honest

- Avoid alcohol

- Avoid drugs

- Not smoke

- Be nice

- Respect others

- Work hard

- Exercise (together!)

You and your friends can also use good peer pressure to help each other resist bad peer pressure. If you see a friend taking some heat, try some of these lines:

- We don't want to drink.

- We don't need to drink to have fun.

- Let's go and do something else.

- Leave her alone. She said she didn't want any.

Chapter 11

Relationships: Friends And Dating

Friendships

Friendships can be tough sometimes. You may be making new friends while still trying to keep old friends. It can also be hard to know what to do when you don't agree with a friend. Keep in mind, you can have a good friendship and still fight sometimes.

Peer Pressure

There are two kinds of peer pressure: positive peer pressure and negative peer pressure. Peer pressure is when you try something because "everyone else is doing it."

Positive peer pressure is when you act a certain way because your friends are acting that way, but it is for a good reason. For example, if your friends talk you into joining the soccer team, and you end up really liking soccer, that's positive peer pressure. Or, if your friend volunteers to tutor younger kids, and you decide you would like to do the same, that's another example of positive peer pressure.

Negative peer pressure is when you feel you have to act a certain way because everyone else is, but the end result is bad. If your friends are mean to the new girl at school and so you treat her badly, too, then that is an example of negative peer pressure.

So why do some teens follow their friends, even when it's not a good idea? Teens may worry about what their friends will think, not know how to say no, or fear being left out. Some

About This Chapter: This chapter begins with information excerpted from "Relationships: Friendships" and "Relationships: Dating," Office on Women's Health (www.girlshealth.gov), September 2009. The chapter concludes with "Understanding Teen Dating Violence," Centers for Disease Control and Prevention (www.cdc.gov), 2012.

friends may pressure you to do something because "everyone else does it," such as making fun of someone, using alcohol or drugs, or smoking. The best thing to do is say, "No, thanks" or "I don't want to." Keep in mind, you are always in charge of what you do and don't do. It can help to talk with your parents or guardians about how to handle pressures that may come up.

Popularity

There are lots of things that you and your friends may do to fit in. It may be having the right clothes or being friends with the cool kids. It is normal to want to be liked by others, but it is more important to focus on what matters to YOU. Having lots of friends and dressing like everyone else may seem important right now, but try to focus on being yourself and having real friends who care about you.

Cliques

A clique is a small group of friends that is very picky about who can and cannot join the group. While it's nice to have a close group of friends, being on the outside of a clique may not be fun. Teens in cliques often leave out other teens on purpose. They may bully kids who are not "cool enough."

If you are being picked on, try to make friends with new people who care about you. Keep in mind, it is the quality or value of the friendship that counts, not how many friends you have. And, if you are leaving someone else out, think about how you would feel if you were the one being left out.

Qualities Of A Good Friend

Here are seven ways to know if your friends really care about you:

- They want you to be happy.
- They listen and care about what you have to say.
- They are happy for you when you do well.
- They say they are sorry when they make a mistake.
- They don't expect you to be perfect.
- They give you advice in a caring way.
- They keep personal things between the two of you.

Source: "Relationships: Friendships," Office on Women's Health (www.girlshealth.gov), September 2009.

There can be a lot of peer pressure in cliques. You may feel like you need to do things like drink or do drugs to be part of the gang. Keep in mind, you always have the right to say no. Real friends will respect that. You also have the right to make new friends.

Bullying

Friendships are very important to adolescents, especially when it comes to having a group of people to hang out with. Sometimes teens compete with each other for friends. When this happens, some kids may leave others out of a circle of friends or even bully them in more open ways. Being left out of a group can really hurt someone's feelings, so think about how what you do makes other people feel. You would want others to include you and treat you nicely.

Making New Friends

It can be really tough when you are meeting a whole bunch of new people at once if you are new at school. You may feel shy or embarrassed. You may feel like you don't have anything to say. But, the other person likely feels the same way. Half the battle is feeling strong enough to talk to new people. And, it will help to just be yourself.

It can also be tough to start hanging around new people at your same school. You may need to do this if you have friends who have been getting into trouble for things like ditching school or doing drugs. Even though you may care about these friends, you have to look out for yourself and make smart choices for you. If you have a hard time breaking away from old friends who may be bad news, talk to a trusted adult for help on how to do your own thing.

Sometimes, you may just want to branch out and meet new people. This is totally okay and you can still keep your old friends. It's easy to hang out with people you've known a long time or have a lot in common with. But, it can also be fun to spend time with new people.

Tips For Handling A Fight With A Friend

In a healthy friendship, you should not be afraid of losing a friend because you say "no." Good friends should respect your right to say no and not give you a hard time. You should show your friends the same respect when they say no to you.

If you and your friend fight about something, it does not mean that you have an unhealthy relationship. You will not always agree with what your friend has to say. But you should always respect one another's ideas. As long as you and your friend listen to what the other has to say, you should be able to work through a fight.

The relationships you have will help you learn a lot about yourself. You will learn about the kind of friends you want to have and the kind of friend you want to be.

Ending A Friendship

Sadly, not all friendships last a lifetime. Sometimes friends grow apart, and sometimes you might need to end a friendship. So how do you know when you should end a friendship?

You should end a friendship if your friend:

- Is sarcastic or mean to you often
- Tells your secrets
- Goes after your crush (or significant other) again and again
- Doesn't want you to have other friends
- Doesn't listen to you
- Pushes you to do dangerous things
- Blames you for what's not good in their lives
- Complains all the time

You could just stop taking your friend's phone calls and stop talking to her at school, but that's not always the best way to end a friendship. The other person may be confused and not understand why you're acting different. A direct talk with the other person may be better. You could try saying, "I feel that you don't listen to me, and friends should support each other." Remember: Honesty is often the best policy.

Dating

Dating relationships can be a fun and exciting part of your life. They can also be confusing, especially if dating is new to you. Once you know that the person that you like also likes you, you may not know what to do next. You can start by learning about what makes a dating relationship healthy and safe.

When do teens start dating?

There is no best age for teens to start dating. Every person will be ready for a dating relationship at a different time. Different families may have their own rules about dating too. When you decide to start a dating relationship, it should be because you care about someone and not because other people are dating. A dating relationship is a special chance to get to know someone, and it should happen only when you are really ready and your parents/guardians are okay with it.

What is a healthy dating relationship?

Healthy dating relationships should start with the same things that healthy friendships start with: good communication, honesty, and respect. Dating relationships are a little different because they may include physical ways of showing you care, like hugging, kissing, or holding hands. You may find yourself wanting to spend all of your time with your crush, but it is important to spend some time apart too. This will let you have a healthy relationship with your crush and with your friends and family at the same time.

Why should I date someone close to my age?

It may not seem like a big deal to date someone more than two years older than you, but it can be. It's possible that someone older than you might want a more physical relationship than you do.

What if I feel pressure to do something I do not want to do?

Respecting your right to say no means that your date will stop if you say "no."

You should never feel pressured to do something that you don't want to do. Your crush should always respect your right to say no to anything that doesn't feel right. Talk to your crush ahead of time about what you will and will not do.

Tips For Having Healthy And Safe Relationships

- Get to know a person by talking on the phone or at school before you go out for the first time.
- Go out with a group of friends to a public place the first few times you go out.
- Plan fun activities like going to the movies or the mall, on a picnic, or for a walk.
- Tell the other person what you feel okay doing. Also, tell the person what time your parents/guardians want you to be home.
- Tell at least one friend and your parents/guardians who you are going out with and where you are going. Also tell them how to reach you.

Communication, trust, and respect are key to healthy relationships. Healthy relationships make you feel good about who you are and safe with the other person. Feel good about yourself, and get to know what makes you happy. The more you love yourself, the easier it will be to find healthy relationships.

Source: "Relationships: Dating," Office on Women's Health (www.girlshealth.gov), September 2009.

Understanding Teen Dating Violence

Dating violence is a type of intimate partner violence. It occurs between two people in a close relationship. The nature of dating violence can be physical, emotional, or sexual.

- **Physical:** This occurs when a partner is pinched, hit, shoved, or kicked.

- **Emotional:** This means threatening a partner or harming his or her sense of self-worth. Examples include name calling, shaming, bullying, embarrassing on purpose, or keeping him/her away from friends and family.

- **Sexual:** This is forcing a partner to engage in a sex act when he or she does not or cannot consent.

- **Stalking:** This refers to a pattern of harassing or threatening tactics used by a perpetrator that is both unwanted and causes fear in the victim.

Dating violence can take place in person or electronically, such as repeated texting or posting sexual pictures of a partner online. Unhealthy relationships can start early and last a lifetime. Dating violence often starts with teasing and name calling. These behaviors are often thought to be a "normal" part of a relationship. But these behaviors can lead to more serious violence like physical assault and rape.

Why is dating violence a public health problem?

Dating violence is a serious problem in the United States. Many teens do not report it because they are afraid to tell friends and family.

- Among adult victims of rape, physical violence, and/or stalking by an intimate partner, 22.4% of women and 15.0% of men first experienced some form of partner violence between 11 and 17 years of age.

- Approximately 9% of high school students report being hit, slapped, or physically hurt on purpose by a boyfriend or girlfriend in the 12 months before surveyed.

How does dating violence affect health?

Dating violence can have a negative effect on health throughout life. Teens who are victims are more likely to be depressed and do poorly in school. They may engage in unhealthy behaviors, like using drugs and alcohol, and are more likely to have eating disorders. Some teens even think about or attempt suicide. Teens who are victims in high school are at higher risk for victimization during college.

How can we prevent dating violence?

The ultimate goal is to stop dating violence before it starts. Strategies that promote healthy relationships are vital. During the preteen and teen years, young people are learning skills they need to form positive relationships with others. This is an ideal time to promote healthy relationships and prevent patterns of dating violence that can last into adulthood.

Prevention programs change the attitudes and behaviors linked with dating violence. One example is Safe Dates, a school-based program that is designed to change social norms and improve problem solving skills.

Who is at risk for dating violence?

Studies show that people who harm their dating partners are more depressed and are more aggressive than peers. Other factors that increase risk for harming a dating partner include:

- Trauma symptoms
- Alcohol use
- Having a friend involved in dating violence
- Having problem behaviors in other areas
- Belief that dating violence is acceptable
- Exposure to harsh parenting
- Exposure to inconsistent discipline
- Lack of parental supervision, monitoring, and warmth

These are just some risk factors. To learn more, go to www.cdc.gov/violenceprevention.

Source: "Understanding Teen Dating Violence: Fact Sheet," Centers for Disease Control and Prevention (www.cdc.gov), 2012.

Chapter 12

Social Phobia

Are you afraid of being judged by others or of being embarrassed all the time? Do you feel extremely fearful and unsure around other people most of the time? Do these worries make it hard for you to do everyday tasks like run errands, or talk to people at work or school?

If so, you may have a type of anxiety disorder called social phobia, also called social anxiety disorder.

What is social phobia?

Social phobia is a strong fear of being judged by others and of being embarrassed. This fear can be so strong that it gets in the way of going to work or school—or doing other everyday things.

Everyone has felt anxious or embarrassed at one time or another. For example, meeting new people or giving a public speech can make anyone nervous but people with social phobia worry about these and other things for weeks before they happen.

People with social phobia are afraid of doing common things in front of other people. For example, they might be afraid to sign a check in front of a cashier at the grocery store, or they might be afraid to eat or drink in front of other people, or use a public restroom. Most people who have social phobia know that they shouldn't be as afraid as they are, but they can't control their fear. Sometimes, they end up staying away from places or events where they think they might have to do something that will embarrass them. For some people, social phobia is a problem only in certain situations, while others have symptoms in almost any social situation.

About This Chapter: Information in this chapter is excerpted from "Social Phobia (Social Anxiety Disorder): Always Embarrassed," National Institute of Mental Health (www.nimh.nih.gov), June 18, 2012.

Social phobia usually starts during youth. A doctor can tell that a person has social phobia if the person has had symptoms for at least six months. Without treatment, social phobia can last for many years or a lifetime.

What causes social phobia?

Social phobia sometimes runs in families, but no one knows for sure why some people have it, while others don't. Researchers have found that several parts of the brain are involved in fear and anxiety. By learning more about fear and anxiety in the brain, scientists may be able to create better treatments. Researchers are also looking for ways in which stress and environmental factors may play a role.

How is social phobia treated?

First, talk to your doctor about your symptoms. Your doctor should do an exam to make sure that another physical problem isn't causing the symptoms. The doctor may refer you to a mental health specialist.

Social phobia is generally treated with psychotherapy, medication, or both.

Psychotherapy: A type of psychotherapy called cognitive behavior therapy is especially useful for treating social phobia. It teaches a person different ways of thinking, behaving, and reacting to situations that help him or her feel less anxious and fearful. It can also help people learn and practice social skills.

Medication: Doctors also may prescribe medication to help treat social phobia. The most commonly prescribed medications for social phobia are anti-anxiety medications and antidepressants. Anti-anxiety medications are powerful and there are different types. Many types begin working right away, but they generally should not be taken for long periods.

Antidepressants are used to treat depression, but they are also helpful for social phobia. They are probably more commonly prescribed for social phobia than anti-anxiety medications. Antidepressants may take several weeks to start working. Some may cause side effects such as headache, nausea, or difficulty sleeping. These side effects are usually not a problem for most people, especially if the dose starts off low and is increased slowly over time. Talk to your doctor about any side effects that you may have.

A type of antidepressant called monoamine oxidase inhibitors (MAOIs) is especially effective in treating social phobia. However, they are rarely used as a first line of treatment because when MAOIs are combined with certain foods or other medicines, dangerous side effects can occur.

What are the signs and symptoms of social phobia?

People with social phobia tend to have these characteristics:

- Be very anxious about being with other people and have a hard time talking to them, even though they wish they could
- Be very self-conscious in front of other people and feel embarrassed
- Be very afraid that other people will judge them
- Worry for days or weeks before an event where other people will be
- Stay away from places where there are other people
- Have a hard time making friends and keeping friends
- Blush, sweat, or tremble around other people
- Feel nauseous or sick to their stomach when with other people

It's important to know that although antidepressants can be safe and effective for many people, they may be risky for some, especially children, teens, and young adults. A "black box"—the most serious type of warning that a prescription drug can have—has been added to the labels of antidepressant medications. These labels warn people that antidepressants may cause some people to have suicidal thoughts or make suicide attempts.

Anyone taking antidepressants should be monitored closely, especially when they first start treatment with medications.

Another type of medication called beta-blockers can help control some of the physical symptoms of social phobia such as excessive sweating, shaking, or a racing heart. They are most commonly prescribed when the symptoms of social phobia occur in specific situations, such as "stage fright."

Some people do better with cognitive behavior therapy, while others do better with medication. Still others do best with a combination of the two. Talk with your doctor about the best treatment for you.

What is it like having social phobia?

"In school I was always afraid of being called on, even when I knew the answers. When I got a job, I hated to meet with my boss. I couldn't eat lunch with my co-workers. I worried about being stared at or judged, and worried that I would make a fool of myself. My heart would pound and I would start to sweat when I thought about meetings. The feelings got worse as the time of the event got closer. Sometimes I couldn't sleep or eat for days before a staff meeting.

I'm taking medicine and working with a counselor to cope better with my fears. I had to work hard, but I feel better. I'm glad I made that first call to my doctor."

Chapter 13

Bullying And Cyberbullying

What Is Bullying?

Aggressive behavior may be bullying depending on what happened, how often it happens and who it happens to.

Bullying Definition

Bullying is unwanted, aggressive behavior among school aged children that involves a real or perceived power imbalance. The behavior is repeated, or has the potential to be repeated, over time. Both kids who are bullied and who bully others may have serious, lasting problems.

In order to be considered bullying, the behavior must be aggressive and include:

- **An Imbalance Of Power:** Kids who bully use their power—such as physical strength, access to embarrassing information, or popularity—to control or harm others. Power imbalances can change over time and in different situations, even if they involve the same people.

- **Repetition:** Bullying behaviors happen more than once or have the potential to happen more than once.

Bullying includes actions such as making threats, spreading rumors, attacking someone physically or verbally, and excluding someone from a group on purpose.

About This Chapter: This chapter begins with excerpts from "What Is Bullying," "Bullying Definition," "The Roles Kids Play," "Effects of Bullying," and "Get Help Now," from StopBullying.gov, a federal government website managed by the U.S. Department of Health and Human Services (www.stopbullying.gov), 2012. Information from the Montana Attorney General's Office about cyberbullying is cited separately within the chapter.

Types Of Bullying

There are three types of bullying:

- Verbal bullying is saying or writing mean things. Verbal bullying includes:
    - Teasing
    - Name-calling
    - Inappropriate sexual comments
    - Taunting
    - Threatening to cause harm

- Social bullying, sometimes referred to as relational bullying, involves hurting someone's reputation or relationships. Social bullying includes:
    - Leaving someone out on purpose
    - Telling other children not to be friends with someone
    - Spreading rumors about someone
    - Embarrassing someone in public

- Physical bullying involves hurting a person's body or possessions. Physical bullying includes:
    - Hitting/kicking/pinching
    - Spitting
    - Tripping/pushing
    - Taking or breaking someone's things
    - Making mean or rude hand gestures

Where And When Bullying Happens

Bullying can occur during or after school hours. While most reported bullying happens in the school building, a significant percentage also happens in places like on the playground or the bus. It can also happen travelling to or from school, in the youth's neighborhood, or on the internet.

Frequency Of Bullying

There are two sources of federally collected data on youth bullying:

- The 2011 Youth Risk Behavior Surveillance System (Centers for Disease Control and Prevention) indicates that, nationwide, 20% of students in grades 9–12 experienced bullying.

- The 2008–2009 School Crime Supplement (National Center for Education Statistics and Bureau of Justice Statistics) indicates that, nationwide, 28% of students in grades 6–12 experienced bullying.

The Roles Kids Play

There are many roles that kids can play. Kids can bully others, they can be bullied, or they may witness bullying. When kids are involved in bullying, they often play more than one role. Sometimes kids may both be bullied and bully others or they may witness other kids being bullied. It is important to understand the multiple roles kids play in order to effectively prevent and respond to bullying.

Importance Of Not Labeling Kids

When referring to a bullying situation, it is easy to call the kids who bully others "bullies" and those who are targeted "victims," but this may have unintended consequences. When children are labeled as "bullies" or "victims" it may:

- Send the message that the child's behavior cannot change

- Fail to recognize the multiple roles children might play in different bullying situations

- Disregard other factors contributing to the behavior such as peer influence or school climate

Instead of labeling the children involved, focus on the behavior. For instance:

- Instead of calling a child a "bully," refer to them as "the child who bullied."

- Instead of calling a child a "victim," refer to them as "the child who was bullied."

- Instead of calling a child a "bully/victim," refer to them as "the child who was both bullied and bullied others."

Kids Involved In Bullying

The roles kids play in bullying are not limited to those who bully others and those who are bullied. Some researchers talk about the "circle of bullying" to define both those directly involved in bullying and those who actively or passively assist the behavior or defend against it. Direct roles include:

- **Kids Who Bully:** These children engage in bullying behavior towards their peers. There are many risk factors that may contribute to the child's involvement in the behavior. Often, these students require support to change their behavior and address any other challenges that may be influencing their behavior.

- **Kids Who Are Bullied:** These children are the targets of bullying behavior. Some factors put children at more risk of being bullied, but not all children with these characteristics will be bullied. Sometimes, these children may need help learning how to respond to bullying.

Even if a child is not directly involved in bullying, they may be contributing to the behavior. Witnessing the behavior may also affect the child, so it is important for them to learn what they should do when they see bullying happen. Roles kids play when they witness bullying include:

- **Kids Who Assist:** These children may not start the bullying or lead in the bullying behavior, but serve as an "assistant" to children who are bullying. These children may encourage the bullying behavior and occasionally join in.

- **Kids Who Reinforce:** These children are not directly involved in the bullying behavior but they give the bullying an audience. They will often laugh or provide support for the children who are engaging in bullying. This may encourage the bullying to continue.

- **Outsiders:** These children remain separate from the bullying situation. They neither reinforce the bullying behavior nor defend the child being bullied. Some may watch what is going on but do not provide feedback about the situation to show they are on anyone's side. Even so, providing an audience may encourage the bullying behavior. (These kids often want to help, but don't know how.)

- **Kids Who Defend:** These children actively comfort the child being bullied and may come to the child's defense when bullying occurs.

Most kids play more than one role in bullying over time. In some cases, they may be directly involved in bullying as the one bullying others or being bullied and in others they may witness bullying and play an assisting or defending role. Every situation is different. Some kids are both bullied and bully others. It is important to note the multiple roles kids play, because:

- Those who are both bullied and bully others may be at more risk for negative outcomes, such as depression or suicidal ideation

- It highlights the need to engage all kids in prevention efforts, not just those who are known to be directly involved

Effects Of Bullying

Bullying can affect everyone—those who are bullied, those who bully, and those who witness bullying. Bullying is linked to many negative outcomes including impacts on mental health, substance use, and suicide. It is important to talk to kids to determine whether bullying—or something else—is a concern.

Kids Who Are Bullied

Kids who are bullied can experience negative physical, school, and mental health issues. Kids who are bullied are more likely to experience:

- Depression and anxiety, increased feelings of sadness and loneliness, changes in sleep and eating patterns, and loss of interest in activities they used to enjoy. These issues may persist into adulthood.

- Health complaints

- Decreased academic achievement—GPA and standardized test scores—and school participation. They are more likely to miss, skip, or drop out of school.

A very small number of bullied children might retaliate through extremely violent measures. In 12 of 15 school shooting cases in the 1990s, the shooters had a history of being bullied.

Kids Who Bully Others

Kids who bully others can also engage in violent and other risky behaviors into adulthood. Kids who bully are more likely to:

- Abuse alcohol and other drugs in adolescence and as adults

- Get into fights, vandalize property, and drop out of school

- Engage in early sexual activity

- Have criminal convictions and traffic citations as adults

- Be abusive toward their romantic partners, spouses, or children as adults

Bystanders

Kids who witness bullying are more likely to:

- Have increased use of tobacco, alcohol, or other drugs

- Have increased mental health problems, including depression and anxiety

- Miss or skip school

The Relationship Between Bullying And Suicide

Media reports often link bullying with suicide. However, most youth who are bullied do not have thoughts of suicide or engage in suicidal behaviors.

Table 13.1. Bullying: Get Help Now

If you have done everything you can to resolve the situation and nothing has worked, or someone is in immediate danger, there are ways to get help.

The Problem	What You Can Do
There has been a crime or someone is at immediate risk of harm.	Call 911.
Someone is feeling hopeless, helpless, thinking of suicide.	Contact the National Suicide Prevention Lifeline at 1-800-273-TALK (800-273-8255).The toll-free call goes to the nearest crisis center in our national network. These centers provide 24-hour crisis counseling and mental health referrals.
Someone is acting differently than normal, such as always seeming sad or anxious, struggling to complete tasks, or not being able care for themselves.	Find a local counselor or other mental health services.
A child is being bullied in school.	Contact the: • Teacher • School counselor • School principal • School superintendent • State Department of Education
The school is not adequately addressing harassment based on race, color, national origin, sex, disability, or religion.	Contact: • School superintendent • State Department of Education • U.S. Department of Education, Office for Civil Rights • U.S. Department of Justice, Civil Rights Division

Source: StopBullying.gov, U.S. Department of Health and Human Services, 2012.

Although kids who are bullied are at risk of suicide, bullying alone is not the cause. Many issues contribute to suicide risk, including depression, problems at home, and trauma history. Additionally, specific groups have an increased risk of suicide, including American Indian and Alaskan Native, Asian American, lesbian, gay, bisexual, and transgender youth. This risk can be increased further when these kids are not supported by parents, peers, and schools. Bullying can make an unsupportive situation worse.

For Teens And Tweens: Cyberbullying

What Is It?

Cyberbullying is "willful and repeated harm inflicted through the use of computers, cell phones, and other electronic devices."

- **Willful:** The actions are deliberate, not accidental.

- **Repeated:** There is a pattern of behavior, not just one isolated incident.

- **Harm:** The target feels hurt or humiliated.

- **Computer, Cell Phones, And Other Electronic Devices:** This is what makes it cyberbullying and not bullying.

Students use technology to bully through personal web pages; social networking sites, such as MySpace, Facebook, or Flickr; YouTube; cell phone, text, picture, and video messages; e-mail and instant messaging (IM'ing); and blogs and forums. Some examples of cyberbullying include:

- "Hot or Not" websites where students rate each other

- Setting up insulting or hateful websites specifically to hurt, tease, embarrass, or humiliate someone

- Hateful or racist e-mail, instant messaging (IM) or text messaging

- Threatening e-mail, IM or text messaging

- Uploading embarrassing or harmful videos or pictures to YouTube, social networking, or other photo- or video-sharing sites without the knowledge of the person or people in the video or picture

- Creating a fake person to carry out embarrassing or hurtful communications or acts on the internet
- Sending repeated messages to a cell phone
- "Borrowing" someone's screen name and pretending to be them while posting a message
- Forwarding private messages, pictures, or video to others

How Common Is It?

A 2008 study found that 72% of students reported being bullied online in the past year.

- Most knew the perpetrator.
- Most often, cyberbullying was done through IM.
- Students who frequently used webcams were the most likely to be repeatedly bullied.
- Insults were the number one reported problem.
- Password theft was the number two reported problem. This involves someone stealing a password, logging onto an account, and sending or uploading content that makes the account owner look bad (Juvonen and Gross, Extending the school grounds?—Bullying experiences in cyberspace, 2008).

Types Of Cyberbullying

- **Cyber Stalking:** Repeatedly sending messages that are threatening or intimidating. Engaging in other online activities that make the victim afraid for his or her safety.
- **Cyber Threats:** The use of a computer, cell phone or other electronic device to threaten a person's physical safety and well-being (Hinduja & Patchin 2009).
- **Defamation:** "Dissing" someone online. Sending or posting cruel gossip or rumors about a person to damage his or her reputation or friendships.
- **Exclusion:** Intentionally excluding someone from an online group, like a buddy list.
- **Flaming Or Trolling:** Online fighting using electronic messages with angry and crude language.
- **Happy Slapping:** A phenomenon that links traditional bullying with cyberbullying where an unsuspected person is recorded being harassed or bullied in a way that usually includes some type of physical abuse. The digital photo or video is uploaded to the web (Hinduja & Patchin 2009).

- **Harassment:** Repeatedly sending offensive, rude, and insulting messages.

- **Impersonation:** Pretending to be someone else and sending or posting material online that makes the victim look bad, gets the victim in trouble or danger, or damages the victim's reputation or friendships.

- **Outing And Trickery:** Sharing someone's secret or embarrassing information online. Tricking someone into revealing secrets or embarrassing information that is then shared online.

- **Photoshopping:** The modification or alteration of a photo or image. This becomes cyberbullying if the image is altered in a humiliating or obscene way and uploaded to the Web (Hinduja & Patchin 2009).

What you may think is funny or a simple prank may not be funny to the victim. The victim may respond very differently than you expect. If you are not sure how the victim of your prank or joke may respond, or if you wouldn't do it to that person's face, then don't do it online. What if you send an embarrassing picture of your girlfriend or boyfriend to a friend, thinking it won't go further than that? The fact is, you have no idea what a friend might do with something you send. Once you have sent it, you have lost control of where it might end up and any harm it might cause. You can get into serious trouble for cyberbullying.

What To Do

To Prevent Cyberbullying

- Don't give out private information (passwords, pins, name, address, phone number, school name, or family and friends' names).

- Don't share your password, even with your friends.

- Don't exchange pictures, videos, or give out e-mail addresses to people you meet online. (Ask for permission from an adult first.)

- Don't share buddy lists.

- Don't send a message when you are angry.

- Don't use profanity or insulting or rude language.

- Delete messages from people you don't know—especially if they seem angry or mean.

- Get out of the site or chat if something doesn't seem right.

- Realize that online conversations are not private.

- Be aware that whatever happens online can be reproduced and spread very easily, by anyone.

- Do not say anything online that you would not say face-to-face to the person on the other end.

If You Are Cyberbullied

- Speak with a trusted adult.

- Speak with your teacher or principal if it is school related.

- Remember that cyberbullying is not about you, it is about bullies who:

  - Want to feel powerful;

  - Are looking for attention; and/or

  - Probably are victims of bullying themselves.

- Don't open or read messages by cyberbullies.

- Don't react to the bully (ignore them).

- Walk away from the computer.

If Ignoring The Bully Doesn't Work?

- Again, speak with a trusted adult or your teacher or principal if it is school related.

- Don't meet with the bully.

- Block the bully.

- Don't erase messages or images from the bully. Instead, save them to a folder as evidence in case the bullying escalates and law enforcement gets involved.

- Contact the internet service provider (ISP) to report the harassment.

- Inform the police if you are threatened with harm.

- Contact the CyberTipline (www.missingkids.com/cybertipline) if:

  - You receive unsolicited obscene material (pornography);

  - You are directed to a misleading domain name (website); or

  - You are tricked into viewing harmful material.

Get Involved

- Develop a Youth Internet Safety Team at your school.

- Become an iMentor and teach your peers or younger students about internet safety (see www.isafe.org to get involved in an iMentor program).

- Teach your parents about what you do while online.

- Teach younger siblings about cyberspace.

- Reach an agreement with your parents about internet rules.

- Consider a Family Internet Use Contract.

Speak Up!

Provide support—be a friend. For example, make positive comments on a friend's Facebook page, especially if others have made negative comments. And let others know that it is not cool to be cruel, to harass someone, or to spread rumors about others. Check out the That's Not Cool website at www.thatsnotcool.com for ideas. Educate your peers and community members about cyberbullying. Here are some ideas from i-SAFE's Student Tool Kit (http://isafe.org):

- Organize a Cyber Safety Week at your school.

- Create PSAs (Public Service Announcements), television, or radio advertisements intended to educate or alert the public on important social issues.

- Set up an information table at lunch, during study hall, at a school sports event, after school, or at the mall or local grocery store to let students, teachers, parents, and community members know about the dangers of cyberbullying.

- Organize a community or school play. This is an ideal activity for school assemblies or a presentation for the class next door or for younger students.

- Organize a Speak Out! (a panel or round table discussion) and ask people to share their experiences or brainstorm strategies for responding to cyberbullying.

- Organize a Pledge Wall for others to write down their pledges to cyber safety.

- Organize a contest for a poster, video, songwriting, poetry, website, or PSA.

- Organize and facilitate a parent training.

- Inspire others to join your efforts by creating media alerts. Start with press releases. Remember, there is strength in numbers.

Chapter 14

Sports Pressure And Competition

Most people play a sport for the thrill of having fun with others who share the same interest. But it's not always fun and games. There can be a ton of pressure in high school sports. A lot of the time it comes from the feeling that a parent or coach expects you to always win.

But sometimes it comes from inside, too: Some players are just really hard on themselves. And individual situations can add to the stress: Maybe there's a recruiter from your number one college scouting you on the sidelines.

Whatever the cause, the pressure to win can sometimes stress you to the point where you just don't know how to have fun anymore.

How can stress affect sports performance?

Stress is a feeling that's created when we react to particular events. It's the body's way of rising to a challenge and preparing to meet a tough situation with focus, strength, stamina, and heightened alertness. A little stress or the right kind of positive stress can help keep you on your toes, ready to rise to a challenge.

The events that provoke stress are called stressors, and they cover a whole range of situations—everything from outright danger to stepping up to take the foul shot that could win the game. Stress can also be a response to change or anticipation of something that's about to happen—good or bad. People can feel stress over positive challenges, like making the varsity team, as well as negative ones.

About This Chapter: "Handling Sports Pressure and Competition," October 2010, reprinted with permission from www.kidshealth.org. This information was provided by KidsHealth®, one of the largest resources online for medically reviewed health information written for parents, kids, and teens. For more articles like this, visit www.KidsHealth.org, or www.TeensHealth.org. Copyright © 1995–2012 The Nemours Foundation. All rights reserved.

Distress is a bad type of stress that arises when you must adapt to too many negative demands. Suppose you had a fight with a close friend last night, you forgot your homework this morning, and you're playing in a tennis match this afternoon. You try to get psyched for the game but can't. You've hit stress overload! Continuous struggling with too much stress can exhaust your energy and drive.

Eustress is the good type of stress that stems from the challenge of taking part in something that you enjoy but have to work hard for. Eustress pumps you up, providing a healthy spark for any task you undertake.

What can I do to ease pressure?

When the stress of competition starts to get to you, try these techniques to help you relax:

- **Deep Breathing:** Find a quiet place to sit down. Inhale slowly through your nose, drawing air deep into your lungs. Hold your breath for about 5 seconds, then release it slowly. Repeat the exercise five times.

- **Muscle Relaxation:** Contract (flex) a group of muscles tightly. Keep them tensed for about 5 seconds, then release. Repeat the exercise five times, selecting different muscle groups.

- **Visualization:** Close your eyes and picture a peaceful place or an event from your past. Recall the beautiful sights and the happy sounds. Imagine stress flowing away from your body. You can also visualize success. People who advise competitive players often recommend that they imagine themselves completing a pass, making a shot, or scoring a goal over and over. Then on game day, you can recall your stored images to help calm nerves and boost self-confidence.

- **Positive Self-Talk:** Watch out for negative thoughts. Whether you're preparing for a competition or coping with a defeat, tell yourself: "I learn from my mistakes!" "I'm in control of my feelings!" "I can make this goal!"

When sports become too stressful, get away from the pressure. Go to a movie or hang out with friends. Put your mind on something completely different.

How can I keep stress in check?

If sports make you so nervous that you get headaches, become nauseated, or can't concentrate on other things, you're experiencing symptoms of unhealthy stress that's becoming a pattern. Don't keep such stress bottled up inside you; suppressing your emotions might mean bigger health troubles for you later on.

Talk about your concerns with a friend. Simply sharing your feelings can ease your anxiety. Sometimes it may help to get an adult's perspective—someone who has helped others deal with sports stress like your coach or fitness instructor. Here are some other things you can do to cope with stress:

- Treat your body right. Eat well and get a good night's sleep, especially before games where the pressure's on.

- Learn and practice relaxation techniques, like those described in the previous section.

- Get some type of physical activity other than the sport you're involved in. Take a walk, ride your bike, and get completely away from the sport that's stressing you out.

- Don't try to be perfect—everyone flubs a shot or messes up from time to time (so don't expect your teammates to be perfect either!). Forgive yourself, remind yourself of all your great shots, and move on.

It's possible that some stress stems only from uncertainty. Meet privately with your coach or instructor. Ask for clarification if his or her expectations seem vague or inconsistent. Although most instructors do a good job of fostering athletes' physical and mental development, you may need to be the one who opens the lines of communication. You may also want to talk with your parents or another adult family member.

If you're feeling completely overscheduled and out of control, review your options on what you can let go. It's a last resort, but if you're no longer enjoying your sport, it may be time to find one that's less stressful. Chronic stress isn't fun—and fun is what sports are all about.

Recognizing when you need guidance to steer yourself out of a stressful situation doesn't represent weakness; it's a sign of courage and wisdom. Don't stop looking for support until you've found it.

Enjoy The Game

Winning is exhilarating! But losing and some amount of stress are part of almost any sports program—as they are in life. Sports are about enhancing self-esteem, building social skills, and developing a sense of community. And above all, sports are about having fun.

Chapter 15

Family Money Troubles

Devon, 17, is used to paying her own cell phone and car expenses. But lately it's been harder. The family she babysits for hasn't been calling as much and she couldn't find a job over the summer. Devon's dad says it's a sign of the tough economy. He told her he's feeling the pinch, too, and that he had to dip into her college fund to pay the mortgage.

These days it's hard to avoid news about the economy. Turn on the computer or TV and words like "recession," "foreclosure," and "unemployment" fill the screen. It can seem a bit scary—and some families are hit really hard.

But as discouraging as things may seem now, the good news is that the economy always gets back on track after a while.

How Does A Difficult Economy Affect Families?

For some people, the slow economy means eating out less or staying home instead of going on vacation. Parents may not have as much money to put toward allowances or college funds. For other families, though, money problems mean bigger changes, such as a parent taking on a second job or the family having to move to a less expensive house.

When a family has money worries, it's easy to get frustrated and upset—and if you feel that way, you're far from alone. Parents also might be more stressed out than usual. They might argue more and worry about how to pay for things.

About This Chapter: "Family Money Troubles," September 2011, reprinted with permission from www.kidshealth .org. This information was provided by KidsHealth®, one of the largest resources online for medically reviewed health information written for parents, kids, and teens. For more articles like this, visit www.KidsHealth.org, or www.TeensHealth.org. Copyright © 1995–2012 The Nemours Foundation. All rights reserved.

Naturally, this can put extra stress on you, too, especially because parents' money problems aren't something you have any control over. But although you can't solve family money troubles, you may find that contributing in some way helps you feel better.

What Can You Do To Make Things Easier?

It's comforting when our lives and routines feel the same, so it's natural to feel worried if things change.

Here are some practical and emotional survival tips for dealing with a tough economy:

- **Think like an entrepreneur.** Jobs may be hard to find, but the slow economy can open up new opportunities. The couple you babysit for might cut back on evenings out, but they could be interested in hiring you for after-school care. Perhaps it's time to hold a yard sale to get rid of the old toys and baby gear in the basement—or help your parents sell these items online. If you're good at navigating online auction sites, you could charge people a fee to sell their old stuff.

- **Prioritize and plan for what you want.** When you want something, write it down. Next to it, write how much you want it on a scale of 1–10. Keep this list going (items may move up or down the scale as you add new ones). Then, figure out a plan to earn any must-have rewards.

- **Talk out troubles.** If you are worried, find a good time and talk to your parents about it. Let them know you can handle the truth. If your parents are fighting, seem stressed, or are sad or angry all the time, talking can really help. If you can't talk to your parents right now, lean on a friend, teacher, or counselor.

- **Practice the art of patience.** Some of your friends might have the latest cell phones, video games, and basketball shoes, but others may be having a tougher time than you. You may not be able to get everything you want, but now is a chance to see if you can master the art of patience without envying friends or feeling negative about your parents.

- **Focus on the positive.** Writing down (or drawing) your frustrations in a journal can be a big step toward dealing with them. But also try to write down three things that you are grateful for each day (or illustrate or write songs if you're more of an artist or composer).

- **Help your friends.** What if a friend is in a really tight spot? Even if you can't think how to help, try just listening: Tell your friend you know it must be hard and that you'll be there for support no matter what. Most friends welcome the chance just to talk through feelings and know that someone understands.

- **Deal with change, but don't burden yourself.** It's good to step in to help friends and family. But it's also good to remind yourself that you're still young and family money troubles are outside your control.

Finding Entertainment On The Cheap

Being creative helps you feel good about yourself at times when life isn't going as you planned, and coming up with free ways to have fun gives your creativity a chance to shine.

Some ways to stay entertained are obvious: Go to the park, ride a bike, take a neighbor's dog for a walk, volunteer, or cook dinner for your friends or family. But why stop there? Think of this as a time to challenge your imagination:

- **Record some music.** If you have a computer and microphone, all you need is your talent.

- **Have a karaoke party.** The worse the singing, the better the fun.

- **Redecorate your room without spending a dime.** Use only stuff you have around the house or found items like shells or old furniture. Discover new uses for old things, like making pillows and lampshades out of old dresses.

- **Learn a new language.** Borrow a "teach-yourself" book or CD from the library.

- **Design your own clothes or jewelry.** Check out thrift stores for clothing you can cut up and customize, or use found items to make jewelry.

- **Plan a surprise picnic for your friends.** Do the whole blanket and picnic basket bit, then find a park or beach and take in the view (and the people watching).

- **Start your own ghost tour.** Check out the creepiest houses in your area and take friends on "haunted house" tours so you can all make up stories about what might have happened there. If you live in a historic town you may be able to research town history and discover enough interesting stories to put together a real tour.

- **Become a caricature artist.** If you're good at art, teach yourself how to draw caricatures. Practice on your family, then when you get better, rent yourself out for children's parties.

- **Host movie night.** Local libraries often loan out movie projectors and movies for free. Get your friends to bring popcorn, pick an upbeat or funny movie, and enjoy!

Eventually the economy will turn around. When it does, you'll be well equipped to deal with any other challenges and difficulties life throws your way!

Chapter 16

Family Violence

What Is Abuse?

Amy's finger was so swollen that she couldn't get her ring off. She didn't think her finger was broken because she could still bend it. It had been a week since her dad shoved her into the wall, but her finger still hurt a lot.

Amy hated the way her dad called her names and accused her of all sorts of things she didn't do, especially after he had been drinking. It was the worst feeling and she just kept hoping he would stop.

Abuse can be physical, sexual, emotional, verbal, or a combination of any or all of these. Abuse can also be neglect, which is when parents or guardians don't take care of the basic needs of the children who depend on them.

Physical Abuse

Physical abuse is often the most easily recognized form of abuse. Physical abuse can be any kind of hitting, shaking, burning, pinching, biting, choking, throwing, beating, and other actions that cause physical injury, leave marks, or cause pain.

About This Chapter: "Abuse," September 2010, is reprinted with permission from www.kidshealth.org. This information was provided by KidsHealth®, one of the largest resources online for medically reviewed health information written for parents, kids, and teens. For more articles like this, visit www.KidsHealth.org. or www.TeensHealth.org. Copyright © 1995–2012 The Nemours Foundation. All rights reserved.

Sexual Abuse

Sexual abuse is any type of sexual contact between an adult and anyone younger than 18; between a significantly older child and a younger child; or if one person overpowers another, regardless of age. If a family member sexually abuses another family member, this is called incest.

Emotional Abuse

Emotional abuse can be the most difficult to identify because there are usually no outward signs of the abuse. Emotional abuse happens when yelling and anger go too far or when parents constantly criticize, threaten, or dismiss kids or teens until their self-esteem and feelings of self-worth are damaged. Emotional abuse can hurt and cause damage just as physical abuse does.

Neglect

Neglect is difficult to identify and define. Neglect occurs when a child or teen doesn't have adequate food, housing, clothes, medical care, or supervision. Emotional neglect happens when a parent doesn't provide enough emotional support or deliberately and consistently pays very little or no attention to a child. This doesn't mean that a parent doesn't give a kid something he or she wants, like a new computer or a cell phone, but refers to more basic needs like food, shelter, and love.

Family violence can affect anyone. It can happen in any kind of family. Sometimes parents abuse each other, which can be hard for a child to witness. Some parents abuse their kids by using physical or verbal cruelty as a way of discipline.

Abuse doesn't just happen in families, of course. Bullying is a form of abusive behavior. Bullying someone through intimidation, threats, or humiliation can be just as abusive as beating someone up. People who bully others may have been abused themselves. This is also true of people who abuse someone they're dating. But being abused is no excuse for abusing someone else.

Abuse can also take the form of hate crimes directed at people just because of their race, religion, abilities, gender, or sexual orientation.

Recognizing Abuse

It may sound strange, but people sometimes have trouble recognizing that they are being abused. Recognizing abuse may be especially difficult for someone who has lived with it for many years. A person might think that it's just the way things are and that there's nothing that can be done. People who are abused might mistakenly think that it's their fault for not doing what their parents tell them, breaking rules, or not living up to someone's expectations.

Growing up in a family where there is violence or abuse can make a person think that is the right way or the only way for family members to treat each other. Somebody who has only known an abusive relationship might mistakenly think that hitting, beating, pushing, shoving, or angry name calling are perfectly normal ways to treat someone when you're mad.

Seeing parents treat each other in abusive ways might lead a child to think that's OK in relationships. But abuse is not a typical or healthy way to treat people.

If you're not sure you are being abused, or if you suspect a friend is, it's always OK to ask a trusted adult or friend.

Why Does Abuse Happen?

If you're one of the thousands of people living in an abusive situation, it can help to understand why some people abuse—and to realize that the abuse is not your fault. Sometimes abusers manipulate those they're abusing by telling them they did something wrong or "asked for it" in some way. But that's not true.

There is no single reason why people abuse others. But some factors seem to make it more likely that someone may lose control, yell, hit, or hurt.

Sometimes, growing up in an abusive family can lead a person to think that example is a good way to discipline others. Others become abusive because they're not able to manage their feelings properly. For example, someone who is unable to control anger or can't cope with stressful personal situations (like the loss of a job or marriage problems) may lash out at others inappropriately. Also, drinking too much and/or drug use can make it difficult for some people to control their actions.

Certain types of personality disorders or mental illness might also interfere with someone's ability to relate to others in healthy ways or cause problems with aggression or self-control. Of course, not everyone with a personality disorder or mental illness becomes abusive.

Fortunately, people who abuse can get help and learn how to take responsibility for how they act—and learn ways to stop.

What Are The Effects Of Abuse?

When people are abused, it can affect every aspect of their lives, especially self-esteem. How much harm is done often depends on the situation and sometimes on how severe the abuse is. Sometimes a seemingly minor thing can trigger a big reaction. Being touched inappropriately by a family member, or being told to keep secrets, for example, can be very confusing and traumatic.

Every family has arguments. Friends, couples, coaches, and teachers can get upset, frustrated, or have a bad day. We all go through difficult times when someone is stressed and angry. Punishments and discipline—like removing privileges, grounding, or being sent to your room—are common.

Yelling and anger can happen in lots of parent-teen relationships and in friendships—although it can feel pretty bad to have an argument with a parent or friend. But if punishments, arguments, or yelling go too far or last too long it can lead to stress and other serious problems.

Teens who are abused (or have been in the past) often have trouble sleeping, eating, and concentrating. They may not do well at school because they are angry or frightened, or feel like they just don't care anymore.

Many people who are abused distrust others. They may feel a lot of anger toward other people and themselves, and it can be hard to make friends. Abuse is a significant cause of depression in young people. Some teens can only feel better by doing things that could hurt them like cutting or abusing drugs or alcohol. They might even attempt suicide.

It's common for those who have been abused to feel upset, angry, and confused about what happened to them. They may feel guilty and embarrassed and blame themselves. But abuse is never the fault of the person who is being abused, no matter how much the abuser tries to blame others.

Abusers may manipulate somebody into keeping quiet by saying stuff like: "This is a secret between you and me," or "If you ever tell anybody, I'll hurt you or your mom," or "You're going to get in trouble if you tell. No one will believe you, and you'll go to jail for lying." This is the abuser's way of making a person feel like nothing can be done so he or she won't report the abuse.

People who are abused might have trouble getting help because it means they'd be reporting on someone they love—someone who may be wonderful much of the time and awful to them only some of the time.

People might be afraid of the consequences of reporting abuse, either because they fear the abuser or the family is financially dependent on that person. For reasons like these, abuse often goes unreported and many kids and teens don't tell anyone what is going on.

What Should Someone Who's Being Abused Do?

People who are being abused need to get help. Keeping the abuse a secret doesn't protect anyone from being abused—it only makes it more likely that the abuse will continue.

If you or anyone you know is being abused, talk to someone you or your friend can trust—a family member, a trusted teacher, a doctor, or a school or religious youth counselor. Many teachers and counselors have training in how to recognize and report abuse.

Telephone and online directories list local child abuse and family violence hotline numbers that you can call for help. There's also Childhelp USA at 800-4-A-CHILD (800-422-4453).

Sometimes people who are being abused by someone in their own home need to find a safe place to live temporarily. It is never easy to have to leave home, but it's sometimes necessary to be protected from further abuse. People who need to leave home to stay safe can find local shelters listed in the phone book or they can contact an abuse helpline. Sometimes a person can stay with a relative or friend.

People who are being abused often feel afraid, numb, or lonely. Getting help and support is an important first step toward feeling better.

Many teens who have experienced abuse find that painful emotions may linger even after the abuse stops. Working with a therapist is one way to sort through the complicated feelings and reactions that being abused creates, and the process can help to rebuild feelings of safety, confidence, and self-esteem.

Chapter 17

When Your Parent Has A Substance Abuse Problem

For Kids And Teens

We know what it's like. You're worried about your mom or dad drinking too much or using other drugs. It's hard to have fun. It's not a family any more. You feel scared and alone. Sad. Ashamed to have friends over. And of course you feel guilty too. Well, don't. You didn't cause it. You can't control it. You can't cure it.

Your parent drinking too much or using drugs is not your fault. (In fact, your mom or dad would drink or use even if you had never been born!) You can't stop it by being good, or by being bad. Your parents still love you, even if the alcohol or drugs makes them unable to show it.

No matter how much you love them or how angry you feel, you cannot make them stop drinking. But you can still feel better about life, and all the things that lie ahead for you.

Is Your Parent's Substance Abuse Your Fault?

No!

Perhaps the most important thing for you to remember is commonly known as the "three C's of addiction":

You didn't <u>C</u>ause it. Addiction is not something that one person can do to another. An unhappy childhood, an unhappy marriage, or problems with children, for example, do not cause a person to become a substance abuser. While some people may be born with an inherited tendency toward addiction, and some life experiences may make it more or less likely, neither genes nor experiences alone cause addiction. Rather, the path to drug use, abuse, and addiction are actions that the substance abuser chooses. Simply stated, the addiction is the result of a series of bad choices made by the substance abuser.

You can't Control it. If an addict wants a drug, nothing and no one will stand in their way. Forget pouring the wine down the sink, or flushing pills down the toilet; it won't make a difference. In truth, the only way to limit being around substance abuse is to limit your time around the substance abuser.

You can't Cure it. Much as you may want a substance abuser to get help, you can't make it happen. Love and understanding won't do it, and neither will begging or threatening. Recovery will come, if at all, only if and when the substance abuser truly decides to seek another life. Just as the addiction was the result of a series of bad choices by the substance abuser, so must recovery begin and be maintained through a series of good choices by the substance abuser.

You cannot control substance abuse, cure it, or cause it. But you can learn to cope with it.

Being Prepared

If your parent has a problem with drugs or alcohol, you should think about having your own personal emergency plan. If you think about this ahead of time, you will be ready if you find yourself in an uncomfortable situation.

- Make sure you know how to call the police, fire department, ambulance service, and doctor. Make sure your brothers and sisters know too.

- Make sure you always have extra money for a phone call, in case it is too dangerous to drive home with a parent who is drunk or high.

- Make up a list of safe places to call for help or to stay—maybe a grandparent, older brother or sister, aunt, uncle, neighbor, or friend. Memorize their phone numbers, and call them if it looks like the situation in your own home might get out of control.

- If you need to study for a big test, or practice your lines for the fall play, ask a neighbor you trust if you can spend some time there, where it is quieter.

- If you want to talk to your mom or dad about the alcohol or drugs, do it when you feel safe and when your parent has not been drinking or using drugs.

Parents With Addiction

You may think you are alone—but you are not. Unfortunately, there are many families across the United States where one of the parents is an alcoholic or drug addict. It is easy to feel like you are the reason why your parent has an alcohol or drug addiction—but that is not true. Nothing you do caused your parent to drink or do drugs. Both are diseases and you need medical attention to overcome them. It is first important to understand the effects the alcohol or drugs will have on your parent. Then you will understand why your parent is acting the way they are.

How does addiction and alcoholism affect my family?

- You may feel a range of emotions from frustrated, to sad, to angry, to lonely, to embarrassed.
- The parent might lose his or her job and might not be able to pay the bills.
- The parent may not be able to care for all the children, and older siblings will have to help take care of younger siblings.
- Some parents are physically or verbally abusive to their children or their spouse.

So what can I do to make the situation better?

- **First, acknowledge that there is a problem.** Don't ignore the problem. The first step to helping your parent is recognizing the problem then speaking to a friend, trusted adult, or a hotline (1-800-344-2666).
- **Recognize your feelings.** Write down your emotions or talk to a friend about them. It is better to voice how you are feeling than bottle it up.
- **Stay informed.** Research alcoholism or drug addiction so you can better understand what your parent's illness is.
- **Stay safe.** If you are avoiding spending time at home because you are afraid, call 800-799-SAFE. This is the National Domestic Violence Hotline. Or, if the danger is immediate, call 911 to get emergency help.
- **Learn the best way to cope**. Your parent may be drinking or doing drugs as a way to cope with problems. However, this is not the correct way to deal with issues. Find a role model that copes through positive activities, such as running or singing.
- **Seek help.** Alcoholics Anonymous and Alateen are groups that provide help for people who are living with alcoholic parents.
- **Finally, stop the cycle.** Because genetics and the environment are important risk factors of alcoholism, children of alcoholic parents are more likely to continue the cycle.

If you are nervous about talking with an adult about what is happening with your parents, ask a friend (who knows the situation) if you can practice with him or her, to help work out ahead of time what you are going to say.

Feeling Better

If you think your parent drinks too much or is addicted to drugs, here is something you should think about: Yourself!

When a parent has a drug or alcohol problem, it's awful. But you are not the only kid in the world who has this trouble. Most people keep alcoholism and drug abuse a secret, but the fact is, there are millions of kids with parents just like yours. They go to your school, live in your neighborhood, and are on your teams and in your clubs. They just don't talk about it—like you probably don't.

What can you do to help yourself feel better?

- Learn the facts about alcohol and other drugs. Just because your parent drinks a lot or uses drugs does not mean that you know the whole truth.

- Talk about it. A lot of kids find that talking about what is happening with a trusted friend or adult makes them feel better. There are probably some people you already know who would be happy to talk with you. Like your teacher, guidance counselor, a relative, doctor, coach, or your best friend. If you don't want to talk to any of these people, you might want to call the people at Alateen. (Alateen is a group of kids like you who meet to talk about their problems.)

- Don't forget to have some fun. Get involved with activities you enjoy—clubs, sports, things that make you feel good about yourself. It doesn't have to be a school activity—maybe you like to laugh with friends or just go out and have fun! In other words, start thinking about yourself. Remember to be a kid!

- Don't use drugs or alcohol yourself. Because your parent has an alcohol or drug problem, you're at higher risk to develop a problem yourself. So be careful!

Chapter 18

Dealing With Divorce

If your parents are recently separated or divorced, you are probably dealing with a lot of changes in your family life. Things may feel like they're changing even if it has been a while since your parents separated or divorced, or if their separation or divorce came as a surprise. You may be living full time with one parent, or you may be going back and forth between both of your parents' homes. You may be living with a parent and your parent's new partner and also dealing with stepbrothers and sisters or new half-brothers and sisters. You may even be living with your grandparents.

Whatever your situation is, it's normal to have many different feelings and emotions about all of these changes. Dealing with divorce or separation can be really hard to get used to, and, as you get older, your feelings may change: Some things may get easier and some things more complicated. This chapter was written to answer the most common questions teens have about coping with divorce and separation.

Ever since my parents told me they're getting divorced, I've been feeling upset all the time. Is this normal?

If your parents are separated, in the process of getting divorced, or recently divorced, it is normal for you to have many complicated feelings. Even if your parents were divorced a while ago, it is still normal to have strong feelings about it. Some common feelings or emotions are:

- Shock or surprise

About This Chapter: Information in this chapter is reprinted from "Dealing With Divorce And Separation," © 2012 Center for Young Women's Health (http://www.youngwomenshealth.org), Boston Children's Hospital. All rights reserved. Used with permission.

- Anxiety (You may worry about what is going to happen to you and who will take care of you and your siblings.)

- Sadness and a feeling of loss

- Anger (You may be angry at your parents or you may feel angry in general.)

- Fear (If one of your parents leaves, you may be afraid of losing your other parent.)

- Guilt (You may feel like it's your fault that your parents split up.)

- Loneliness (You may feel that you have no one to talk to or that no one understands what you are going through.)

- Worry (You may worry about whether you will have a good relationship or marriage in the future.)

- Embarrassment (You may not want anyone to know that things are going to be different in your family.)

You may also feel relieved (because there is less stress at home) and happy to have special time alone with each parent.

All of these feelings are a normal part of coping with all of the changes in your family life. If these feelings are making you feel overwhelmed and upset, it would be best for you to talk with your parents, a trusted adult, or a friend. Holding your feelings in will not make them go away! Many teens who are going through a family divorce find it helpful to talk with a counselor or therapist too.

Your health care provider should be able to help you find a specially trained person such as a social worker or psychologist to talk to about your family situation. There may be someone at your school who is available to meet with you, and some schools even have groups for students who are coping with new situations. Talking with someone can help you feel better while you're dealing with difficult times, and it can also help you to find solutions to problems that you may not have thought of on your own.

Remember
- It's normal to have strong feelings (ranging from anger to relief) about your parents' divorce.
- Ask both of your parents to be open with you so you know what to expect.
- It's helpful to talk with a counselor to help you cope with your feelings.

I'm relieved that my parents got divorced. Is this normal?

Sometimes when parents get divorced they do so after a lot of arguing or fighting, or sometimes your parents may have appeared to not be speaking to each other at all. In some families there may even have been physical violence, alcohol problems, or other situations that created stress in the home. After the divorce or separation, it is normal to feel relieved that your home life has become less stressful and more stable. This is nothing to feel guilty about! Your parents may also feel relieved even though they may also feel badly about not being together.

Since my parents got divorced, nothing in my life is the same. Will it always be this hard?

After a divorce, your everyday life can feel confusing. It may not seem like it now, but dealing with all of the changes will get easier with time. The many changes that come with divorce are hard to accept all at once. You will need time to think about things and adjust to changes as they come about, and figure out what works best for you and each of your parents in your new lives together. It can help to have someone to talk to about what you're going through. It's especially important that you understand that it is NOT your fault that your parents are getting separated or divorced.

Here are some of the ways divorce might change your life:

- Custody arrangements and visitations—you may only be able to see or stay with your parents on certain days that were decided by your parents a mediator, a lawyer, and/or the court;

- Your parents may be sad, preoccupied or upset for a while after the divorce;

- You probably won't see one of your parents as much as you did before the divorce;

- You may have trouble concentrating in school;

- You may have to move and you may have to change schools;

- You may have a different relationship with your grandparents, aunts and uncles, cousins, or other family members as they, too, get used to the changes;

- One or both of your parents may be dating; and/or

- Your family finances may be strained.

These changes can be a lot to deal with at first, but it will get easier, over time, if you talk with your parents about how the changes are affecting you.

My parents don't get along, and I always feel like I'm in the middle. How can I tell them what would make this situation easier on me?

There are many things parents can do to try to make life easier after a divorce. You may want to share the following tips with your parents:

- It's best if both parents stay involved with you and reassure you that they will always love and care for you. If one of your parents moves away or does not stay in touch, it is not your fault.

- It's important for parents to try not to put you in the middle. Sometimes your parents may be tempted to complain about each other or have you deliver messages back and forth. This may make you feel like you have to choose between your parents or that you are not being loyal enough to one of your parents. If this is happening, it's okay to tell a parent that their behavior upsets you.

- It's important for your parents to try to get along, especially about things that directly affect you, like visits, school issues, holidays and other things that need to be discussed.

- It's best for you to have as few changes as possible, at least for a while. Sometimes it may be necessary to move and/or to go to a new school. You may be unhappy about these familiar things changing too! If this has to happen, tell your parents that you would like to be able to stay in touch with your friends from your old neighborhood and school.

Even if your parents try their best to make things easier for you, they may not be able to do all of these things all of the time. Remember that your parents are also trying to deal with the changes in their marriage as well as in your family life. They may not always be as tuned in to your needs as they were before. Learning how to express your feelings to your parents will really help to let them know what's important to you.

My parents got divorced when I was little. Shouldn't I have gotten over it by now?

If your parents got divorced when you were younger, you may have gotten used to some of the changes more easily, and in some ways feel comfortable with your parents not being together. However, you may still have many strong feelings about the divorce, even though other people think you have gotten over it. This is normal, because as you have grown older, you may be more aware of how the divorce shaped your family. You may have questions for your parents and ask for more age-appropriate explanations. Also, as you get older, the visitation and vacation arrangements may no longer work because of your social or school activities. It's important to talk to your parents when you think it is time to change your arrangements, and try to work with them to figure out a new schedule that fits your life and theirs.

What are some ways I can deal with stress?

There are many ways to relieve stress. Some teens write in journals or listen to music; some play sports, read, draw, or talk to friends. If your usual ways of dealing with stress are not helping, you may want to talk to a school guidance counselor, mental health professional, or clergy person.

Separation and divorce can cause new situations as time goes on, for example, if your mom or dad—or both—get remarried. You may also have to adjust to having step-brothers or sisters, or even a new baby. As these new situations come up, it's normal to have new feelings about your parent's divorce. Remember that although divorce can complicate your life, in time you will learn how to handle your new family situations.

Chapter 19

Stepfamily Stress

Sometimes when parents break up, or someone passes away, mom or dad may eventually start a new relationship. This is how people come to have stepfamilies. All relationships have their ups and downs, and stepfamilies are no exception. When one or more people join your family, it can create a lot of change and this can be hard to accept at first—but being in a stepfamily can be really cool too.

Benefits Of Stepfamilies

There are many good things about living in a stepfamily.

- Some young people have said they like the idea of being a "family" again.

- Others say that they feel more safe and secure.

- Some young people have said they have two sets of parents to look up to, to get support from, to help with homework, to talk with about other problems, and to help with major decisions (e.g., education and career).

- You have another adult to do things with.

- You may have stepbrothers and sisters to do things with and have fun.

- Some may enjoy the differences between two homes.

- Some say it's nice to see their parent so happy being with a new partner.

About This Chapter: "Step-Families," reprinted with permission from Women's and Children's Health Network (www.cyh.com) © 2011 Government of South Australia.

- Some young people recognize that their standard of living is better because there is more money coming into the household.

- Having more relatives can be positive.

- There may be a new baby brother or sister to love.

- Some have said that one benefit is getting more presents!

- Others enjoy having a bigger family.

The "Not-So-Good" Stuff

Being in a stepfamily may not always be fun. There can be some difficult issues to deal with. The following sections cover some of the potential problems, and how they can be worked through.

Loss

Young people in new stepfamilies will have experienced important losses, [such as]:

- You may have been through the trauma of your parents breaking up and experienced all the feelings of loss this brings.

- When one parent moves into another relationship, this can mean the loss of all your dreams and wishes that your parents will reunite.

- If a parent has died, there is grief and mourning for the loss of your parent.

- There may be the loss of time and attention from your parent as she spends time in the new relationship.

- There is a loss of the old familiar ways of how your family used to be and the ways that the family used to do things.

- If stepbrothers and sisters move in, it may mean having to give up or share your bedroom.

- If you're moving to a new house, it may mean the loss of a familiar neighborhood, friends, and school.

Just one of these losses alone can be difficult to deal with; yet sometimes young people will have to face several losses at one time.

When this happens, support and love from parents is really comforting. Sometimes parents can be caught up in what is happening for themselves with the breakup, death, or the new relationship, and need time for themselves also.

- Try talking to your parents about how you are feeling; ask for help and share the new experiences together.

- Try working out solutions together (e.g., if you are moving, can arrangements be made for you to stay at your old school?).

- If it's too hard to talk to your parents, is there a relative or adult family friend you trust and can talk to?

- How about your student counselor, teacher, or youth health service?

Change

In a new stepfamily, young people have to get used to different ways of doing things and get used to living with new people. Apart from the new stepparent, there may be new stepbrothers and stepsisters to get used to. For example:

- You might not be the oldest or the youngest in the family anymore.

- Change can also be a source of stress, and even simple changes such as day-to-day chores around the house can take time to get used to, [for example]:

  - Do you do the dishes after each meal of the day or do you do them once a day?

  - What meal times and routines are people used to?

  - Do you eat meals at the table or in front of the television?

  - How do you divide up household tasks?

Change can also be a good thing. You might learn new and better ways of doing things in a stepfamily, or you might be able to teach other members of the stepfamily some new ideas.

Feeling Torn

Some young people feel like they're divided between their two natural parents.

- You may love both parents, but feel bad because there is still some conflict between them. It can be really upsetting to hear awful things about the other parent.

- You could notice one parent is still really upset about the breakup. The breakup probably happened for many reasons, not just one thing, and neither person can be entirely to blame. All you can do is let the hurting parent know that you love him or her and that you care, and maybe do something nice for that parent.

- As hard as it is for you, these things are for your parents to work out. It is their problem. If you're angry about the break up, it can be best to find other ways to get the anger out, perhaps by talking to a school counselor.

- Some parents continually ask young people questions about the other parent. It's best not to get involved. You may have to even tell your parent, "I don't want to get involved telling you things about Mom (or about Dad). It is too hard for me to be pulled in the middle. If you want to know things, please ask her (or him)." Say it as respectfully, yet as assertively, as you can manage.

- Sometimes a parent may say things about the other parent which make you feel bad. Maybe you could say something like, "I know you're upset, so let's talk about something else."

Discipline

It can be difficult to get used to the idea of discipline coming from a stepparent.

- Your new stepparent may have different ideas about discipline from your parent.

- If the issue becomes a problem, it's best to get things out into the open and let your parent know how you are feeling.

  - The most effective way to discuss any conflict is to make a time to talk together when you won't be interrupted.

  - Be respectful and try and stay calm. (Yes, it is difficult when you're upset about something, but it works better this way.)

- If you can't talk to your parent, is there a family friend or relative who can help? Is there a school counselor who can help?

Moving Between Houses

Sometimes young people can have two houses to stay at. If things aren't going well at one, then it's handy to have somewhere else to go to. But if this becomes a way to avoid solving problems, then house hopping can become a problem in itself. An alternative to constantly moving between houses might be:

- Tell your parent/s you want to discuss something that is really important to you and ask that they make a time when you can sit down together quietly.

  - Tell them how you're feeling—in a respectful way, without blaming.

- Ask if there is any way you can work this out together (e.g., set new rules that give you a little more freedom, so that you all know exactly where you stand).

- If [talking to your parent/s] is just too hard, is there a relative you could talk to who could speak to your parents for you?

- Would you consider going to counseling or mediation with your parents? Mediation is when a trained person helps both parties to come to an agreement together. The mediator should not take sides.

Getting Kicked Out

Sometimes it happens that there is so much conflict between a young person and parent or stepparent that the parents ask or demand that the young person leave the home. If this happens, it is a good idea to check out where you stand by talking to someone at your local government body responsible for children's welfare.

- In most places parents do have some responsibility for their children, depending on their age.

- There are counseling services that can help to mediate the situation.

- If the conflict can't be resolved, can you live with another family member? Can you stay with a family member for a while so that you and your parents can have a break from each other?

Contact

Contact refers to the time young people and parents agree to share with one another. Contact can have its ups and downs.

Some of the good things are having fun with your other parent, going out with him/her, seeing other relatives or stepbrothers and stepsisters, and talking with (and getting support from) your parent.

Some of the tougher things can be living out of a suitcase, and feeling like it's not really your home. See if you can make it more like home for yourself. Here are some ideas:

- Ask if you can put up a poster or two.

- Keep some of your "things" there, like a trophy or something you made at school.

- Ask if you can have a cupboard or even a drawer you can keep things in.

- Keep a toothbrush and a few spare clothes there.

- Can you invite a friend over?

- Can you give the phone number to your friends so they can call you there?

- Try and keep up with your usual weekend sports—if your parent or stepparent can't take you, can you arrange something else?

Stepparents

You don't have to like your stepparent—although it would be nicer for you both if you do like each other. It can be difficult living in the same house with an adult you don't like. The best way to ensure that things run smoothly in the home is if everyone tries to treat everyone else with respect.

Many stepparents feel unsure of themselves and their place in the family; they can feel like outsiders. [Here are ways you can help:]

- You could try doing some nice things for your stepparent to include her in the family. Little things like saying thanks for a ride or a meal can be helpful; so can saying hello goodbye as you would with your parent.

- Inviting a stepparent to your sports grand final or another function can be helpful in including them in your family life.

Stepparents seem to take on different roles.

- Some are like friends, some are like another parent and others seem like a distant stranger.

- There's no real right or wrong; it's what works best for your family and the different people who are in your family.

Some stepparents get really bossy and try to take control of everything. It is hard to get along with someone who is bossy all the time. In this situation, it may be best to get counseling or mediation [in order] to live together in a more positive way.

Sometimes it can be so tough, young people start using drugs and alcohol as a way to try and forget painful feelings.

- This may work for a short time while the person is affected by a drug, but doesn't always block the bad feelings out (think about people who get drunk and cry about their problems).

- When the person straightens up, the problems and painful feelings are still there because the feelings haven't really been dealt with.

- What's worse, you may have spent a ton of money, have a hangover, or have taken other health, legal and safety risks in using drugs.

It's best to get some support about ways to handle the feelings. That way you'll find solutions that last. Talk to a counselor or another supportive friend or relative.

If A Stepparent Is Abusive

If you are in a situation of real abuse from a stepparent or a parent, this is very different from the normal (but still difficult) conflicts that arise in a family. It is important to get some outside help.

Step Siblings

Sometimes stepbrothers and stepsisters get along really well and become close friends. Sometimes they become friends for life.

Sometimes stepbrothers and stepsisters become sexually attracted to each other. It is normal to become attracted to someone you like. But in a stepfamily it can become a problem for several reasons.

- Having a relationship with someone in the same household can cause all kinds of upset to relationships in the house.

- Parents may suspect young people of sneaking into each other's bedrooms and arguments begin between parents and the young people.

- The couple may argue or break up (which is highly likely at a young age) and this can cause major dramas in the household.

- One may eventually want to go out with another person. Can you imagine how uncomfortable that other person would feel coming over to the house?

What is the answer? It can be difficult to handle this attraction. It may be best to bring the situation out into the open by talking about it to your parents or to speak to a counselor a school, a youth service, or a community health center.

Chapter 20

Moving

Moving is a big decision. There can be many reasons why you (or your family) are moving. It could be that you want to move out to be more independent or because you have to study or work in another city. You may have to leave home because you don't get along with your parents, or the whole family may be moving. Sometimes parents move without their children. You could be moving from the city to the country, interstate, or overseas. Whatever the reason or the location, it involves a lot of planning and careful thought.

Whether you choose to move or have to, it can involve a major life change. Sometimes we are able to plan things, other times we have to act quickly. Be prepared!

Be Prepared

As moving can mean different things to different people, there are a lot of questions you can ask yourself and the people around you:

- What will this mean for me?

- Why do I want to move out?

- How will Mom and Dad take this?

- Where will I go?

- What can I afford?

- How will I move?

About This Chapter: "Moving," reprinted with permission from Women's and Children's Health Network (www.cyh.com) © 2011Government of South Australia.

- What do my friends think?

- What will this mean for my relationship/school/work?

- How will I cope?

- When is the best time?

- What are my rights?

- Where can I get support?

- Can I come home if I need to?

- Will I be close to the things/people I need?

If you are moving with your family here are some questions for you:

- Why does the family have to move?

- How does everyone feel about the move?

- Where will we go?

- How will I cope?

- How are we going to move?

- Do I want to stay behind or go with them?

- What will my friends think?

- Will I have to change schools?

- What are the new opportunities for me?

- What are the benefits of living somewhere new?

Positives And Negatives

There will always be positives and negatives in every major change you make in your life. Thinking about the advantages and positives will help you to be inspired about the move and to get the most out of the situation. Understanding the disadvantages will help so that you can be prepared and plan the change as best you can. Many positives and negatives can be the same depending on the way you view the situation, the reasons behind the move, and your support system. Some of the positives include:

- Freedom
- Independence
- Individuality
- Sense of identity
- Ability to make your own decisions
- New experiences
- Change of scenery
- Get along better with parents
- More responsibility
- Less conflict
- New friendships and relationships
- Confidence in yourself

Some of the negatives could include:

- Conflict with family
- Stress on the family
- Losing touch with friends
- Relationships ending
- Changing schools
- Losing part time work
- Losing the day to day contact with your family
- More responsibility
- Having to remember to pay the bills yourself
- Losing some practical things such as a television, use of the family car, etc.
- Lack of support

Note: If you are moving because your parents have to move because of work, you may feel very upset or cross about having to leave your friends. Tell your parents how you feel so you can work out together the best way to cope with the change. You may be able to visit old friends or have them to visit after the move, to phone them in the evenings when the rates are lower, or to correspond by e-mail.

Remember that you have good skills to make friends because you already have friends that you are leaving, but don't expect too much too soon—it takes time. Joining in with sport or clubs at your new home, as soon as you can, will help you make the most of every possibility. There is always some sadness at times of change as well as new challenges and opportunities. Trying to make the most of it, even if you did not want to go, is the best way to enjoy your new life—and you will end up with friends in two or more places, not just one!

Your Parents

If you're leaving home, or staying behind when your family moves, you may have to deal with your parents' reaction/feelings about your decision. Having a child leave home (no matter what the young person's age) can be a difficult transition for parents to make; after all, you have been a major part of their lives for a lot of years. The way parents react can vary considerably. Some parents may see it as positive and accept your need for independence; others may be concerned about your ability to manage or your safety; while others may think you're leaving because you don't like to follow the rules at home, or because you don't like them. Reactions will be different based upon the relationship you had with your parents before you made this decision.

If you have a good relationship with your family/parents you will probably want to sit down and discuss the situation. Try to do this before you make any definite plans. Be clear about what you want to do (and why), so you can best explain this to your parents. Listen to their views, and try to understand where they're coming from. Let them know you appreciate their concern and respect their views. Try to work the issue through as a team. (Think about using a problem solving technique.)

It may also make your parents feel better if they can be involved in your planning, or if you propose a trial period (this could work well for you too!).

Going It Alone

If you're going to rent an apartment or house, by yourself or with a friend, consider the following things:

- Rights and responsibilities—both for yourself and the landlord or real estate agent. Take note of the conditions of your lease and your obligations. Get some advice if you're unsure—speak to your local rental assistance or tenancy authority.

- Make sure you inspect the property, taking note of things that are damaged or needing repair. Bring these to the attention of your landlord or agent before you sign an agreement. Keep a written copy signed by all parties concerned; in fact keep copies of all the paperwork involved.

- Take someone with you when you look—you may not notice something but your friend might! Keep in mind the types of facilities available, safety and security, and the location and position of the premises for convenience to transport, etc. See if you can negotiate things like security doors before you move in.

- Check out how quickly repairs will be made, when necessary, and if things can be done after hours in an emergency.

- Look at your budget. Work out how much you can afford, when rent is due, and take note of what you need to get started.

Leaving Home After Conflict

Some of you may not have a choice about leaving home. You may be escaping conflict or violence, or living in a difficult family situation. Moving because you have been asked to leave can be very stressful and you will probably need as much support as possible.

If your situation is difficult, and you have been unable to resolve the conflict at home, you need to find yourself a safe place to stay. **Remember, your physical and emotional safety is very important!**

If you have to move in a hurry, consider the following support systems:

- Friends, other family members, or a trusted neighbor
- Your local police station (especially if you are under 18 years of age)
- Your local community health center

Keeping In Contact—Coping With The Move

Often, when you move, you can lose touch with family or friends. Most people are so busy getting settled in that they have no time to think about how they will keep in contact with the people most important to them. Try to work this out with family and friends before you move. Exchange phone numbers, e-mail, and home addresses, or arrange to get together on a regular basis.

If you're moving out of home, you may like to get together with your family once a week for a meal. Invite them to your place sometimes. Try to also be around for special occasions like birthdays. Family and friends can be the most supportive, so keeping in contact is important.

If you are moving a long way from family and friends, look for supports in your new area (this can be something you look at when planning your move). Youth services or community centers often provide support to young people. You may also want to join a club or youth network to make new friends and to develop interests in your new location. Keeping busy and meeting new people will also help you to avoid feeling sad and will allow you to get used to your new environment.

Remember, it takes time to adjust to new surroundings. It takes time to settle in and get used to a new place. If you allow yourself the time to adjust, you will feel less pressure and more comfortable with the changes you have made.

Part Three
Effects Of Stress On The Body, Mind, And Behavior

Chapter 21

Effects Of Childhood Stress On Health Across The Lifespan

Stress is an inevitable part of life. Human beings experience stress early, even before they are born. A certain amount of stress is normal and necessary for survival. Stress helps children develop the skills they need to cope with and adapt to new and potentially threatening situations throughout life. Support from parents and/or other concerned caregivers is necessary for children to learn how to respond to stress in a physically and emotionally healthy manner.

The beneficial aspects of stress diminish when it is severe enough to overwhelm a child's ability to cope effectively. Intensive and prolonged stress can lead to a variety of short- and long-term negative health effects. It can disrupt early brain development and compromise functioning of the nervous and immune systems. In addition, childhood stress can lead to health problems later in life including alcoholism, depression, eating disorders, heart disease, cancer, and other chronic diseases. The purpose of this chapter is to summarize the research on childhood stress and its implications for adult health and well-being.

Types Of Stress

Following are descriptions of the three types of stress that The National Scientific Council on the Developing Child has identified based on available research:

Positive Stress: Positive stress results from adverse experiences that are short-lived. This type of stress causes minor physiological changes including an increase in heart rate and

---

About This Chapter: Information in this chapter is excerpted from "The Effects of Childhood Stress on Health across the Lifespan," Centers for Disease Control and Prevention (www.cdc.gov), 2008. Reviewed by David A. Cooke, MD, FACP, April 2013.

changes in hormone levels. With the support of caring adults, children can learn how to manage and overcome positive stress. This type of stress is considered normal and coping with it is an important part of the development process.

Tolerable Stress: Tolerable stress refers to adverse experiences that are more intense but still relatively short-lived. Examples include the death of a loved one, a natural disaster, a frightening accident, and family disruptions such as separation or divorce.

Toxic Stress: Toxic stress results from intense adverse experiences that may be sustained over a long period of time—weeks, months, or even years. As a result, the stress response system gets activated for a prolonged amount of time. This can lead to permanent changes in the development of the brain.

The Effects Of Toxic Stress On Brain Development In Early Childhood

The ability to manage stress is controlled by brain circuits and hormone systems that are activated early in life. When a child feels threatened, hormones are released and they circulate throughout the body. Prolonged exposure to stress hormones can impact the brain and impair functioning in a variety of ways.

- Toxic stress can impair the connection of brain circuits and, in the extreme, result in the development of a smaller brain.

- Brain circuits are especially vulnerable as they are developing during early childhood. Toxic stress can disrupt the development of these circuits. This can cause an individual to develop a low threshold for stress, thereby becoming overly reactive to adverse experiences throughout life.

- High levels of stress hormones, including cortisol, can suppress the body's immune response. This can leave an individual vulnerable to a variety of infections and chronic health problems.

- Sustained high levels of cortisol can damage the hippocampus, an area of the brain responsible for learning and memory. These cognitive deficits can continue into adulthood.

The National Scientific Council on the Developing Child has been studying the effects of toxic stress on brain development. Papers summarizing the scientific literature can be found on-line at www.developingchild.net.

Stress And Disease: What's The Connection?

Doctors have pondered the connection between our mental and physical health for centuries. Until the 1800s, most believed that emotions were linked to disease and advised patients to visit spas or seaside resorts when they were ill. Gradually emotions lost favor as other causes of illness (such as bacteria or toxins) emerged, and new treatments such as antibiotics cured illness after illness.

More recently, scientists have speculated that even behavioral disorders, such as autism, have a biological basis. At the same time, they have been rediscovering the links between stress and health. Today, we accept that there is a powerful mind-body connection through which emotional, mental, social, spiritual, and behavioral factors can directly affect our health.

Mind-body medicine focuses on treatments that may promote health, including relaxation, hypnosis, visual imagery, meditation, yoga, and biofeedback.

Over the past 20 years, mind-body medicine has provided evidence that psychological factors can play a major role in such illnesses as heart disease, and that mind-body techniques can aid in their treatment. Clinical trials have indicated mind-body therapies to be helpful in managing arthritis and other chronic pain conditions. There is also evidence they can help to improve psychological functioning and quality of life, and may help to ease symptoms of disease.

Source: Excerpted from "Emotions and Health," *The Mind-Body Connection*, National Institutes of Health (www.nih.gov), 2008. Reviewed by David A. Cooke, MD, FACP, April 2013.

The Effects Of Toxic Stress On Adult Health And Well-Being

Research findings demonstrate that childhood stress can impact adult health. The Adverse Childhood Experiences (ACE) Study is particularly noteworthy because it demonstrates a link between specific 1) violence–related stressors, including child abuse, neglect, and repeated exposure to intimate partner violence, and 2) risky behaviors and health problems in adulthood.

The ACE Study

The ACE Study, a collaboration between the Centers for Disease Control and Prevention (CDC) and Kaiser Permanente's Health Appraisal Clinic in San Diego, uses a retrospective approach to examine the link between childhood stressors and adult health. Over 17,000 adults participated in the research, making it one of the largest studies of its kind. Each participant completed a questionnaire that asked for detailed information on their past history of abuse, neglect, and family dysfunction as well as their current behaviors and health status. Researchers were particularly interested in participants' exposure to the following ten ACE:

Abuse

- Emotional
- Physical
- Sexual

Neglect

- Emotional
- Physical

Household Dysfunction

- Mother treated violently
- Household substance abuse
- Household mental illness
- Parental separation or divorce
- Incarcerated household member

General ACE Study Findings

The ACE Study findings have been published in more than 30 scientific articles. The following are some of the general findings of the study:

- Childhood abuse, neglect, and exposure to other adverse experiences are common. Almost two-thirds of study participants reported at least one ACE, and more than one in five reported three or more.

- The short- and long-term outcomes of ACE include a multitude of health and behavioral problems. As the number of ACE a person experiences increases, the risk for the following health outcomes also increases:

  - Alcoholism and alcohol abuse
  - Chronic obstructive pulmonary disease
  - Depression

- Fetal death

- Illicit drug use

- Ischemic heart disease

- Liver disease

- Risk for intimate partner violence

- Multiple sexual partners

- Sexually transmitted diseases

- Smoking

- Suicide attempts

- Unintended pregnancies

- ACE are also related to risky health behaviors in childhood and adolescence, including pregnancies, suicide attempts, early initiation of smoking, sexual activity, and illicit drug use.

- As the number of ACE increases, the number of co-occurring health conditions increases.

Violence-Related ACE Study Findings

Findings from the ACE Study confirm what we already know—that too many people in the United States are exposed early on to violence and other childhood stressors. The study also provides strong evidence that being exposed to certain childhood experiences, including being subjected to abuse or neglect or witnessing intimate partner violence (IPV), can lead to a wide array of negative behaviors and poor health outcomes. In addition, the ACE Study has found associations between experiencing ACE and two violent outcomes: suicide attempts and the risk of perpetrating or experiencing IPV.

The Link Between ACE And Suicide Attempts

- Almost four percent (3.8%) of study participants reported having attempted suicide at least once.

- Experiencing one ACE increased the risk of attempted suicide two to five times.

- As the ACE score increased so did the likelihood of attempting suicide.

- The relationship between ACE and the risk of attempted suicide appears to be influenced by alcoholism, depression, and illicit drug use.

ACE And Associated Health Behaviors

Associations were found between ACE and many negative health behaviors. A partial list of behaviors is included below. For a complete list, see the ACE Study web site at www.cdc .gov/nccdphp/ace/index.htm.

- Participants with higher ACE scores were at greater risk of alcoholism.

- Those with higher ACE scores were more likely to marry an alcoholic.

- Study participants with higher ACE scores were more likely to initiate drug use and experience addiction.

- Those with higher ACE scores were more likely to have 30 or more sexual partners, engage in sexual intercourse earlier, and feel more at risk of contracting AIDS.

- Higher ACE scores in participants were linked to a higher probability of both lifetime and recent depressive disorders.

Chapter 22

Stress And Your Immune System

What The Research Shows

Stressed out? Lonely or depressed? Don't be surprised if you come down with something. Psychologists in the field of "psychoneuroimmunology" have shown that state of mind affects one's state of health.

In the early 1980s, psychologist Janice Kiecolt-Glaser, PhD, and immunologist Ronald Glaser, PhD, of the Ohio State University College of Medicine, were intrigued by animal studies that linked stress and infection. From 1982 through 1992, these pioneer researchers studied medical students. Among other things, they found that the students' immunity went down every year under the simple stress of the three-day exam period. Test takers had fewer natural killer cells, which fight tumors and viral infections. They almost stopped producing immunity-boosting gamma interferon and infection-fighting T-cells responded only weakly to test-tube stimulation.

Those findings opened the floodgates of research. By 2004, Suzanne Segerstrom, PhD, of the University of Kentucky, and Gregory Miller, PhD, of the University of British Columbia, had nearly 300 studies on stress and health to review. Their meta-analysis discerned intriguing patterns. Lab studies that stressed people for a few minutes found a burst of one type of "first responder" activity mixed with other signs of weakening. For stress of any significant duration—from a few days to a few months or years, as happens in real life—all aspects of immunity went downhill. Thus long-term or chronic stress, through too much wear and tear, can ravage the immune system.

The meta-analysis also revealed that people who are older or already sick are more prone to stress-related immune changes. For example, a 2002 study by Lyanne McGuire, PhD, of John Hopkins School of Medicine with Kiecolt-Glaser and Glaser reported that even chronic, sub-clinical mild depression may suppress an older person's immune system. Participants in the study were in their early 70s and caring for someone with Alzheimer's disease. Those with chronic mild depression had weaker lymphocyte-T cell responses to two mitogens, which model how the body responds to viruses and bacteria. The immune response was down even 18 months later, and immunity declined with age. In line with the 2004 meta-analysis, it appeared that the key immune factor was duration, not severity, of depression. And in the case of the older caregivers, their depression and age meant a double-whammy for immunity.

The researchers noted that lack of social support has been reported in the research as a risk factor for depression, an insight amplified in a 2005 study of college students. Health psychologists Sarah Pressman, PhD, Sheldon Cohen, PhD, and fellow researchers at Carnegie Mellon University's Laboratory for the Study of Stress, Immunity, and Disease, found that social isolation and feelings of loneliness each independently weakened first-year students' immunity.

In the study, students got flu shots at the university health center, described their social networks, and kept track of their day-to-day feelings using a handheld computer (a new technique called "momentary ecological awareness"). They also provided saliva samples for measuring levels of the stress hormone cortisol. Small networks and loneliness each independently weakened immunity to a core vaccine component. Immune response was most weakened by the combination of loneliness and small social networks, an obvious health stress facing shy new students who have yet to build their friendship circles.

What The Research Means

Emerging evidence is tracing the pathways of the mind-body interaction. For example, as seen with the college students, chronic feelings of loneliness can help to predict health status—perhaps because lonely people have more psychological stress or experience it more intensely and that stress in turn tamps down immunity. It's also no surprise that depression hurts immunity; it's also linked to other physical problems such as heart disease. At the same time, depression may both reflect a lack of social support and/or cause someone to withdraw from social ties. Both can be stressful and hurt the body's ability to fight infection.

What Is The Immune System?

The immune system is a network of cells, tissues, and organs that work together to defend the body against attacks by "foreign" invaders. These are primarily microbes—tiny organisms such as bacteria, parasites, and fungi that can cause infections. Viruses also cause infections, but are too primitive to be classified as living organisms. The human body provides an ideal environment for many microbes. It is the immune system's job to keep them out or, failing that, to seek out and destroy them.

When the immune system hits the wrong target, however, it can unleash a torrent of disorders, including allergic diseases, arthritis, and a form of diabetes. If the immune system is crippled, other kinds of diseases result.

The immune system is amazingly complex. It can recognize and remember millions of different enemies, and it can produce secretions (release of fluids) and cells to match up with and wipe out nearly all of them.

The secret to its success is an elaborate and dynamic communications network. Millions and millions of cells, organized into sets and subsets, gather like clouds of bees swarming around a hive and pass information back and forth in response to an infection. Once immune cells receive the alarm, they become activated and begin to produce powerful chemicals. These substances allow the cells to regulate their own growth and behavior, enlist other immune cells, and direct the new recruits to trouble spots.

Although scientists have learned much about the immune system, they continue to study how the body launches attacks that destroy invading microbes, infected cells, and tumors while ignoring healthy tissues. New technologies for identifying individual immune cells are now allowing scientists to determine quickly which targets are triggering an immune response. Improvements in microscopy are permitting the first-ever observations of living B cells, T cells, and other cells as they interact within lymph nodes and other body tissues.

In addition, scientists are rapidly unraveling the genetic blueprints that direct the human immune response, as well as those that dictate the biology of bacteria, viruses, and parasites. The combination of new technology and expanded genetic information will no doubt reveal even more about how the body protects itself from disease.

Source: From "Immune System: What Is the Immune System?" National Institute of Allergy and Infectious Diseases (www.niaid.nih.gov), December 19, 2011.

All of these findings extend what we know about how stress management and interpersonal relationships can benefit day-to-day health, doing everything from helping us combat the common cold to speeding healing after surgery. The research is in synch with anecdotal reports of how people get sick in stressful times, but understanding exactly how psychology affects biology helps scientists to recommend the best ways we can build up immunity.

How We Use The Research

Managing stress, especially chronic or long-term stress (even if it's not intense), may help people to fight germs. When burdened with long-term stressors, such as caring for an elderly parent or spouse with dementia, health can benefit from conscientious stress management.

Kiecolt-Glaser and Glaser confirmed this hopeful option by comparing the immune function of exam-stressed medical students given hypnosis and relaxation training with that of students without training. At first, the immune responses of the two groups appeared to both go down. However, closer inspection revealed that some students took this exercise more seriously than others. Those who didn't take relaxation training seriously didn't fare so well; those who practiced conscientiously did actually have significantly better immune function during exams than students who practiced erratically or not at all.

Finally, the newest findings on social stress underscore the value of good friends; even just a few close friends can help someone feel connected and stay strong. Social ties may indirectly strengthen immunity because friends—at least health-minded friends—can encourage good health behaviors such as eating, sleeping, and exercising well. Good friends also help to buffer the stress of negative events.

The Immune System And The Nervous System

Evidence is mounting that the immune system and the nervous system are linked in several ways. One well-known connection involves the adrenal glands. In response to stress messages from the brain, the adrenal glands release hormones into the blood. In addition to helping a person respond to emergencies by mobilizing the body's energy reserves, these "stress hormones" can stifle the protective effects of antibodies and lymphocytes.

Another link between the immune system and the nervous system is that the hormones and other chemicals that convey messages among nerve cells also "speak" to cells of the immune system. Indeed, some immune cells are able to manufacture typical nerve cell products, and some lymphokines can transmit information to the nervous system. Moreover, the brain may send messages directly down nerve cells to the immune system. Networks of nerve fibers have been found connecting to the lymphoid organs.

Source: From "Immune System: The Immune System and the Nervous System," National Institute of Allergy and Infectious Diseases (www.niaid.nih.gov), February 25, 2009.

Chapter 23

Can Stress Cause Cancer?

Psychological stress alone has not been found to cause cancer, but psychological stress that lasts a long time may affect a person's overall health and ability to cope with cancer. Therefore, people who are better able to cope with stress have a better quality of life while they are being treated for cancer—but they do not necessarily live longer.

What is psychological stress?

Psychological stress describes what people feel when they are under mental, physical, or emotional pressure. Although it is normal to experience some psychological stress from time to time, people who experience high levels of psychological stress or who experience it repeatedly over a long period of time may develop health problems (mental and/or physical).

Stress can be caused both by daily responsibilities and routine events, as well as by more unusual events, such as a trauma or illness in oneself or a close family member. When people feel that they are unable to manage or control changes caused by cancer or normal life activities, they are in distress. Distress has become increasingly recognized as a factor that can reduce the quality of life of cancer patients. There is even some evidence that extreme distress is associated with poorer clinical outcomes. Clinical guidelines are available to help doctors and nurses assess levels of distress and help patients manage it.

About This Chapter: Information in this chapter is excerpted from "Psychological Stress and Cancer," National Cancer Institute (www.cancer.gov), December 2012.

How does the body respond during stress?

The body responds to physical, mental, or emotional pressure by releasing stress hormones (such as epinephrine and norepinephrine) that increase blood pressure, speed heart rate, and raise blood sugar levels. These changes help a person act with greater strength and speed to escape a perceived threat.

Research has shown that people who experience intense and long-term (i.e., chronic) stress can have digestive problems, fertility problems, urinary problems, and a weakened immune system. People who experience chronic stress are also more prone to viral infections such as the flu or common cold and to have headaches, sleep trouble, depression, and anxiety.

Can psychological stress cause cancer?

Although stress can cause a number of physical health problems, the evidence that it can cause cancer is weak. Some studies have indicated a link between various psychological factors and an increased risk of developing cancer, but others have not.

Apparent links between psychological stress and cancer could arise in several ways. For example, people under stress may develop certain behaviors, such as smoking, overeating, or drinking alcohol, which increase a person's risk for cancer. Or someone who has a relative with cancer may have a higher risk for cancer because of a shared inherited risk factor, not because of the stress induced by the family member's diagnosis.

How does psychological stress affect people who have cancer?

People who have cancer may find the physical, emotional, and social effects of the disease to be stressful. Those who attempt to manage their stress with risky behaviors such as smoking or drinking alcohol or who become more sedentary may have a poorer quality of life after cancer treatment. In contrast, people who are able to use effective coping strategies to deal with stress, such as relaxation and stress management techniques, have been shown to have lower levels of depression, anxiety, and symptoms related to the cancer and its treatment. However, there is no evidence that successful management of psychological stress improves cancer survival.

Evidence from experimental studies does suggest that psychological stress can affect a tumor's ability to grow and spread. For example, some studies have shown that when mice bearing human tumors were kept confined or isolated from other mice—conditions that increase stress—their tumors were more likely to grow and spread (metastasize). In one set of experiments, tumors transplanted into the mammary fat pads of mice had much higher rates of spread to the lungs and lymph nodes if the mice were chronically stressed than if the mice were not stressed. Studies in mice and in human cancer cells grown in the laboratory have found that the stress hormone norepinephrine, part of the body's fight-or-flight response system, may promote angiogenesis and metastasis.

In another study, women with triple-negative breast cancer who had been treated with neoadjuvant chemotherapy (treatment given as a first step to shrink a tumor) were asked about their use of beta blockers, which are medications that interfere with certain stress hormones, before and during chemotherapy. Women who reported using beta blockers had a better chance of surviving their cancer treatment without a relapse than women who did not report beta blocker use. There was no difference between the groups, however, in terms of overall survival.

Although there is still no strong evidence that stress directly affects cancer outcomes, some data do suggest that patients can develop a sense of helplessness or hopelessness when stress becomes overwhelming. This response is associated with higher rates of death, although the mechanism for this outcome is unclear. It may be that people who feel helpless or hopeless do not seek treatment when they become ill, give up prematurely on or fail to adhere to potentially helpful therapy, engage in risky behaviors such as drug use, or do not maintain a healthy lifestyle, resulting in premature death.

How can people who have cancer learn to cope with psychological stress?

Emotional and social support can help patients learn to cope with psychological stress. Such support can reduce levels of depression, anxiety, and disease- and treatment-related symptoms among patients. Approaches can include the following:

- Training in relaxation, meditation, or stress management
- Counseling or talk therapy
- Cancer education sessions
- Social support in a group setting
- Medications for depression or anxiety
- Exercise

Some expert organizations recommend that all cancer patients be screened for distress early in the course of treatment. A number also recommend re-screening at critical points along the course of care. Health care providers can use a variety of screening tools, such as a distress scale or questionnaire, to gauge whether cancer patients need help managing their emotions or with other practical concerns. Patients who show moderate to severe distress are typically referred to appropriate resources, such as a clinical health psychologist, social worker, chaplain, or psychiatrist.

Chapter 24

Stress And Your Developing Brain

The Teen Brain: Still Under Construction

One of the ways that scientists have searched for the causes of mental illness is by studying the development of the brain from birth to adulthood. Powerful new technologies have enabled them to track the growth of the brain and to investigate the connections between brain function, development, and behavior.

The research has turned up some surprises, among them the discovery of striking changes taking place during the teen years. These findings have altered long-held assumptions about the timing of brain maturation. In key ways, the brain doesn't look like that of an adult until the early 20s.

An understanding of how the brain of an adolescent is changing may help explain a puzzling contradiction of adolescence: Young people at this age are close to a lifelong peak of physical health, strength, and mental capacity, and yet, for some, this can be a hazardous age. Mortality rates jump between early and late adolescence. Rates of death by injury between ages 15 to 19 are about six times that of the rate between ages 10 and 14. Crime rates are highest among young males and rates of alcohol abuse are high relative to other ages. Even though most adolescents come through this transitional age well, it's important to understand the risk factors for behavior that can have serious consequences. Genes, childhood experience, and the environment in which a young person reaches adolescence all shape behavior. Adding to this complex picture, research is revealing how all these factors act in the context of a brain that is changing, with its own impact on behavior.

About This Chapter: Information for this chapter is excerpted from "The Teen Brain: Still Under Construction," National Institute of Mental Health (www.nimh.nih.gov), May 2012.

The more we learn, the better we may be able to understand the abilities and vulnerabilities of teens, and the significance of this stage for life-long mental health.

The "Visible" Brain

A clue to the degree of change taking place in the teen brain came from studies in which scientists did brain scans of children as they grew from early childhood through age 20. The scans revealed unexpectedly late changes in the volume of gray matter, which forms the thin, folding outer layer or cortex of the brain. The cortex is where the processes of thought and memory are based. Over the course of childhood, the volume of gray matter in the cortex increases and then declines. A decline in volume is normal at this age and is in fact a necessary part of maturation.

The assumption for many years had been that the volume of gray matter was highest in very early childhood and gradually fell as a child grew. The more recent scans, however, revealed that the high point of the volume of gray matter occurs during early adolescence.

While the details behind the changes in volume on scans are not completely clear, the results push the timeline of brain maturation into adolescence and young adulthood. In terms of the volume of gray matter seen in brain images, the brain does not begin to resemble that of an adult until the early 20s.

The scans also suggest that different parts of the cortex mature at different rates. Areas involved in more basic functions mature first: those involved, for example, in the processing of information from the senses and in controlling movement. The parts of the brain responsible for more "top-down" control, controlling impulses, and planning ahead—the hallmarks of adult behavior—are among the last to mature.

What's Gray Matter?

The details behind the increase and decline in gray matter are still not completely clear. Gray matter is made up of the cell bodies of neurons, the nerve fibers that project from them, and support cells. One of the features of the brain's growth in early life is that there is an early blooming of synapses—the connections between brain cells or neurons—followed by pruning as the brain matures. Synapses are the relays over which neurons communicate with each other and are the basis of the working circuitry of the brain. Already more numerous than an adult's at birth, synapses multiply rapidly in the first months of life. A two-year-old has about half again as many synapses as an adult.

Scientists believe that the loss of synapses as a child matures is part of the process by which the brain becomes more efficient. Although genes play a role in the decline in synapses, animal research has shown that experience also shapes the decline. Synapses "exercised" by experience survive and are strengthened, while others are pruned away. Scientists are working to determine to what extent the changes in gray matter on brain scans during the teen years reflect growth and pruning of synapses.

A Spectrum Of Change

Research using many different approaches is showing that more than gray matter is changing:

- Connections between different parts of the brain increase throughout childhood and well into adulthood. As the brain develops, the fibers connecting nerve cells are wrapped in a protein that greatly increases the speed with which they can transmit impulses from cell to cell.

- Several lines of evidence suggest that the brain circuitry involved in emotional responses is changing during the teen years. Functional brain imaging studies, for example, suggest that the responses of teens to emotionally loaded images and situations are heightened relative to younger children and adults.

- Enormous hormonal changes take place during adolescence. Reproductive hormones shape not only sex-related growth and behavior, but overall social behavior. Hormone systems involved in the brain's response to stress are also changing during the teens. As with reproductive hormones, stress hormones can have complex effects on the brain, and as a result, behavior.

- In terms of sheer intellectual power, the brain of an adolescent is a match for an adult's. The capacity of a person to learn will never be greater than during adolescence. At the same time, behavioral tests, sometimes combined with functional brain imaging, suggest differences in how adolescents and adults carry out mental tasks. Adolescents and adults seem to engage different parts of the brain to different extents during tests requiring calculation and impulse control, or in reaction to emotional content.

- Research suggests that adolescence brings with it brain-based changes in the regulation of sleep that may contribute to teens' tendency to stay up late at night. Along with the obvious effects of sleep deprivation, such as fatigue and difficulty maintaining attention, inadequate sleep is a powerful contributor to irritability and depression. Studies of children and adolescents have found that sleep deprivation can increase impulsive behavior;

Does Stress Affect Your Developing Brain?

It is well known that the early months and years of life are critical for brain development. But the question remains: Just how do early influences act on the brain to promote or challenge the developmental process? Research has suggested that both positive and negative experiences, chronic stressors, and various other environmental factors may affect a young child's developing brain. And now, studies involving animals are revealing in greater detail how this may occur.

One important line of research has focused on brain systems that control stress hormones—cortisol, for example. Cortisol and other stress hormones play an important role in emergencies: They help our bodies make energy available to enable effective responses, temporarily suppress the immune response, and sharpen attention. However, a number of studies conducted in people with depression indicate that excess cortisol released over a long time span may have any negative consequences for health. Excess cortisol may cause shrinking of the hippocampus, a brain structure required for the formation of certain types of memory.

In experiments with animals, scientists have shown that a well-defined period of early postnatal development may be an important determinant of the capacity to handle stress throughout life. Striking differences were seen in rat pups removed from their mothers for periods of three hours a day, a model of maternal neglect, compared to pups that were not separated. After three hours, the mother rats tended to ignore the pups—at least initially—upon their return. In sharp contrast to those pups that were greeted attentively by their mothers after a short absence, the "neglected" pups were shown to have a more profound and excessive stress response in subsequent tests. This response appeared to last into adulthood.

The implications of these animal studies are worrisome. However, research is in progress to determine the extent to which the hypersensitive or dysregulated stress response of "neglected" rat pups can be reversed if, for example, foster mothers are provided who will groom the pups more intensely, or if the animals are raised in an "enriched" environment following their separation. An enriched setting may include, for example, a diverse and varied diet, a running wheel, mazes, and changes of toys.

Animal investigators are well aware of another kind of long-term change, again rooted in the first days of life. Laboratory rats are often raised in shoebox cages with few sources of stimulation. Scientists have compared these animals to rats raised in an enriched environment and found that the "privileged" rats consistently have a thicker cerebral cortex and denser networks of nerve cells than the "deprived" rats.

It is far too early to draw firm conclusions from these animal studies about the extent to which early life experience produces a long-lived or permanent set point for stress responses, or influences the development of the cerebral cortex in humans. However, animal models that show the interactive effect of stress and brain development deserve serious consideration and continued study.

Source: Excerpted from "Stress and the Developing Brain," National Institute of Mental Health (www.nimh.nih.gov), January 2001. Reviewed by David A. Cooke, MD, FACP, April 2013.

some researchers report finding that it is a factor in delinquency. Adequate sleep is central to physical and emotional health.

The Changing Brain And Behavior In Teens

One interpretation of all these findings is that, in teens, the parts of the brain involved in emotional responses are fully online, or even more active than in adults, while the parts of the brain involved in keeping emotional, impulsive responses in check are still reaching maturity. Such a changing balance might provide clues to a youthful appetite for novelty and a tendency to act on impulse—without regard for risk.

The Adolescent And Adult Brain

It is not surprising that the behavior of adolescents would be a study in change, since the brain itself is changing in such striking ways. Scientists emphasize that the fact that the teen brain is in transition doesn't mean it is somehow not up to par. It is different from both a child's and an adult's in ways that may equip youth to make the transition from dependence to independence. The capacity for learning at this age, an expanding social life, and a taste for exploration and limit testing may all, to some extent, be reflections of age-related biology.

Understanding the changes taking place in the brain at this age presents an opportunity to intervene early in mental illnesses that have their onset at this age.

Chapter 25

Stress Affects Mental Health

Stress—Frequently Asked Questions

Stress—just the word may be enough to set your nerves on edge. Everyone feels stressed from time to time. Some people may cope with stress more effectively or recover from stressful events quicker than others. It's important to know your limits when it comes to stress to avoid more serious health effects.

What is stress?

Stress can be defined as the brain's response to any demand. Many things can trigger this response, including change. Changes can be positive or negative, as well as real or perceived. They may be recurring, short-term, or long-term and may include things like commuting to and from school or work every day, traveling for a yearly vacation, or moving to another home.

Changes can be mild and relatively harmless, such as winning a race, watching a scary movie, or riding a rollercoaster. Some changes are major, such as marriage or divorce, serious illness, or a car accident. Other changes are extreme, such as exposure to violence, and can lead to traumatic stress reactions.

How does stress affect the body?

Not all stress is bad. All animals have a stress response, which can be life-saving in some situations. The nerve chemicals and hormones released during such stressful times, prepares the

About This Chapter: This chapter is excerpted from "Adult Stress—Frequently Asked Questions," National Institute of Mental Health (www.nimh.nih.gov), March 2013; "Anxiety Disorders," U.S. Department of Health and Human Services, Office on Women's Health (www.womenshealth.gov) April 2010; and "Depression," National Institute of Mental Health (www.nimh.nih.gov), June 2012.

animal to face a threat or flee to safety. When you face a dangerous situation, your pulse quickens, you breathe faster, your muscles tense, your brain uses more oxygen and increases activity—all functions aimed at survival. In the short term, it can even boost the immune system.

However, with chronic stress, those same nerve chemicals that are life-saving in short bursts can suppress functions that aren't needed for immediate survival. Your immunity is lowered and your digestive, excretory, and reproductive systems stop working normally. Once the threat has passed, other body systems act to restore normal functioning. Problems occur if the stress response goes on too long, such as when the source of stress is constant, or if the response continues after the danger has subsided.

How does stress affect your overall health?

There are at least three different types of stress, all of which carry physical and mental health risks, including: routine stress related to the pressures of school, family, and other daily responsibilities; stress brought about by a sudden negative change; and traumatic stress, experienced in an event like a major accident, war, assault, or a natural disaster where one may be seriously hurt or in danger of being killed.

The body responds to each type of stress in similar ways. Different people may feel it in different ways. For example, some people experience mainly digestive symptoms, while others may have headaches, sleeplessness, depressed mood, anger, and irritability. People under chronic stress are prone to more frequent and severe viral infections, such as the flu or common cold, and vaccines, such as the flu shot, are less effective for them.

Anxiety Disorders

What is anxiety?

Anxiety is a normal reaction to stress. It helps you deal with a tense situation, study harder for an exam, or keep focused on an important speech. In general, it helps you cope. But when anxiety becomes an excessive, irrational dread of everyday things, it can be disabling.

Anxiety disorders are not the same as the mild stress you may feel when you have to speak in public or the butterflies you may feel in your stomach when going on a first date. Anxiety disorders can last at least six months and can get worse if they are not treated.

What is generalized anxiety disorder (GAD)?

All of us worry about things like health, money, or family problems at one time or another. But people with GAD are extremely worried about these and many other things, even when there is little or no reason to worry about them. They may be very anxious about just getting through the day. They think things will always go badly. At times, worrying keeps people with GAD from doing everyday tasks. People with GAD tend to worry very much about everyday things (for at least six months, even if there is little or no reason to worry about them); can't control their constant worries; know that they worry much more than they should; can't relax; have a hard time concentrating; are easily startled; and may have trouble falling asleep or staying asleep.

GAD may also affect the body. Common symptoms may include feeling tired for no reason; headaches; muscle tension and aches; having a hard time swallowing; trembling or twitching; being irritable; sweating; nausea; feeling lightheaded; feeling out of breath; having to go to the bathroom a lot; and hot flashes.

GAD develops slowly—during the time between childhood and middle age. Symptoms may get better or worse at different times, and often are worse during times of stress.

People with GAD may visit a doctor many times before they find out they have this disorder. They ask their doctors to help them with the signs of GAD, such as headaches or trouble falling asleep, but don't always get the help they need right away. It may take doctors some time to be sure that a person has GAD instead of something else.

Treatment For Generalized Anxiety Disorder

If you think you have an anxiety disorder such as GAD, the first person you should see is your family doctor. A physician can determine whether the symptoms that alarm you are due to an anxiety disorder, another medical condition, or both.

Early treatment can help keep the disease from progressing to its later stages, and people can learn effective ways to live with this disorder. Treatment options include: medications, cognitive therapy, behavioral therapy, or a combination of these treatments.

Source: Excerpted from "Generalized Anxiety Disorder," U.S. Department of Health and Human Services, Office on Women's Health (www.womenshealth.gov), March 2010.

What is panic disorder?

People with panic disorder have sudden attacks of terror. These attacks include: a pounding heart, sweatiness, weakness, faintness, dizziness, feeling overly warm or chilled, tingling or numb hands, and/or nausea, chest pain, or smothering sensations.

Panic attacks usually produce a sense of unreality, a fear of impending doom, or a fear of losing control. A fear of one's own unexplained physical symptoms is also a sign of panic disorder. People having panic attacks sometimes believe they are having heart attacks, losing their minds, or are dying. They can't predict when or where an attack will occur, and between episodes, many worry a lot and fear the next attack.

Panic attacks can occur at any time, even during sleep. An attack usually peaks within 10 minutes, but some symptoms may last much longer.

People who have full-blown, repeated panic attacks can become very disabled by their condition and should seek treatment before they start to avoid places or situations where panic attacks have occurred. For example, if a panic attack happened in an elevator, someone with panic disorder may develop a fear of elevators that could affect the choice of a job or an apartment. This fear could also restrict where that person can seek medical attention or enjoy entertainment.

What is post-traumatic stress disorder (PTSD)?

PTSD starts after a scary ordeal that involved physical harm or the threat of physical harm. The person who develops PTSD may have been the one who was harmed, the harm may have happened to a loved one, or the person may have witnessed a harmful event that happened to loved ones or strangers.

PTSD can cause many symptoms. These symptoms can be grouped into three categories:

- **Re-Experiencing Symptoms:** May cause problems in a person's everyday routine. They can start from the person's own thoughts and feelings. Words, objects, or situations that are reminders of the event can also trigger symptoms, including flashbacks, bad dreams, and/or frightening thoughts.

- **Avoidance Symptoms:** Things that remind a person of the traumatic event can trigger avoidance symptoms. These symptoms may cause a person to change his or her personal routine, including: staying away from places, events, or objects that are reminders of the experience; feeling emotionally numb; feeling strong guilt, depression, or worry; losing interest in things that were enjoyable in the past; and/or having trouble remembering the dangerous event.

- **Hyperarousal Symptoms:** Symptoms are usually constant and may make it hard to do daily tasks, such as sleeping, eating, or concentrating. Hyperarousal symptoms include: being easily startled, feeling tense or "on edge," having difficulty sleeping; and/or having angry outbursts.

It's normal to have some of these symptoms after a dangerous event. Sometimes people have very serious symptoms that go away after a few weeks. This is called acute stress disorder, or ASD.

When the symptoms last more than a few weeks and become an ongoing problem, they might be PTSD. Some people with PTSD don't show any symptoms for weeks or months.

What is social phobia (social anxiety disorder)?

Social phobia, also called social anxiety disorder, is diagnosed when people become very anxious and self-conscious in everyday social situations. People with social phobia have a strong fear of being watched and judged by others. They embarrass easily.

Social phobia can happen in one kind of situation, such as talking to people, eating or drinking, or writing on a blackboard in front of others. Or, it may be so broad that the person experiences anxiety around almost anyone other than family members.

Physical symptoms may include: blushing, profuse sweating, trembling, nausea, and/or difficulty talking. When these symptoms occur, people with social phobia feel as though everyone is watching them.

What are some common specific phobias?

A specific phobia is an intense, irrational fear of something that poses little or no actual danger. Some of the more common specific phobias are fears of closed-in places, heights, escalators, tunnels, highway driving, water, flying, dogs, and injuries involving blood. These fears are irrational. For example, you may be able to ski the world's tallest mountains with ease but be unable to go above the fifth floor of an office building. Adults with phobias know that these fears are irrational but they often find that facing, or even thinking about facing, their fears brings on a panic attack or severe anxiety.

Treatment For Panic Disorder

If you think you have an anxiety disorder such as panic disorder, the first person you should see is your family doctor. A physician can determine whether the symptoms that alarm you are due to an anxiety disorder, another medical condition, or both.

Early treatment can help keep the disease from getting worse, and people can learn effective ways to live with this disorder. Treatment options include: medications, cognitive therapy, behavioral therapy, or a combination of these treatments.

Source: Excerpted from "Panic Disorder," U.S. Department of Health and Human Services, Office on Women's Health (www.womenshealth.gov), March 2010.

Can anxiety disorders be treated?

Yes, there are treatments that can help people with anxiety disorders. There is no cure for anxiety disorder yet, but treatments can give relief to people who have it and help them live a more normal life. The first step is to go to a doctor or health clinic to talk about your symptoms. The doctor will do an exam to make sure that another physical problem isn't causing the symptoms. The doctor may make a referral to a mental health specialist.

Doctors may prescribe medication to help relieve anxiety disorders. It's important to know that some of these medicines may take a few weeks to start working. In most states only a medical doctor (a family doctor or psychiatrist) can prescribe medications.

Doctors also may ask people with anxiety disorders to go to talk therapy with a licensed social worker, psychologist, or psychiatrist. This treatment can help people with anxiety disorders feel less anxious and fearful. If you know someone with signs of an anxiety disorder, talk to him or her about seeing a doctor. Offer to go along for support.

What can I do to help myself if I have an anxiety disorder?

Many people find it helps to join a support group because they can share their problems and successes with others who are going through the same thing. Internet chat rooms can be useful for support, but any advice received over the Internet should be used with caution. Internet friends may have never seen each other, and false identities are common.

While it doesn't take the place of mental health care, talking with trusted friends or a member of your faith community can also be very helpful. Family members can play an important role in a person's treatment by offering support. Learning how to manage stress will help you to stay calm and focused. Research suggests that aerobic exercise (like jogging, bicycling, and swimming) may be calming. Other studies have found that caffeine, illegal drugs, and some over-the-counter cold medicines can worsen the symptoms of these disorders. Check with your doctor or pharmacist before taking any over-the-counter medicines.

Where can I find help for my anxiety disorder?

If you don't know where to go for help, talk to someone you trust who has experience in mental health—for example, a doctor, nurse, social worker, or religious counselor. Ask their advice on where to seek treatment. If there is a university nearby, its departments of psychiatry or psychology may offer private and/or sliding-scale- fee clinic treatment options. In times of crisis, the emergency room doctor at a hospital may be able to provide temporary help for a mental health problem and will be able to tell you where and how to get further help.

Obsessive Compulsive Disorder

People with obsessive compulsive disorder (OCD) have thoughts (obsessions) or rituals (compulsions) which happen over and over again. Rituals—such as hand washing, counting, checking on a specific item (like whether the oven was left on), or cleaning—often are done in hope of stopping the thoughts. Doing these rituals, though, gives only short-term relief. Ignoring the urge to do the ritual greatly increases anxiety. Left untreated, obsessions and the need to perform rituals can take over a person's life. OCD is often a chronic, relapsing illness.

People with OCD sometimes have other mental health disorders, such as depression, eating disorders, substance abuse, attention deficit hyperactivity disorder (ADHD), or other anxiety disorders. When a person also has other disorders, OCD is often harder to diagnose and treat. A person can have symptoms of OCD at the same time as, or that are part of, other brain disorders, such as Tourette's syndrome. Getting the right diagnosis and treatment of other disorders is important to successful treatment of OCD.

Treatment

If you think you have obsessive compulsive disorder, the first person you should see is your family doctor. A physician can determine whether the symptoms that alarm you are due to an anxiety disorder, another medical condition, or both.

Research shows that people with OCD have patterns of brain activity that differ from people with other mental illnesses or people with no mental illness at all. There is also proof that both behavioral therapy and medication can help people with OCD. A type of behavioral therapy known as "exposure and response prevention" is very useful for treating OCD. In this approach, a person is exposed to whatever triggers the obsessive thoughts, and then is taught ways to avoid doing the compulsive rituals and how to deal with the anxiety.

Source: Excerpted from "Mental Health: Obsessive Compulsive Disorder," U.S. Department of Health and Human Services, Office on Women's Health (www.womenshealth.gov), March 2010.

Depression

What is depression?

Everyone occasionally feels blue or sad. But these feelings are usually short-lived and pass within a couple of days. When you have depression, it interferes with daily life and causes pain for both you and those who care about you. Depression is a common but serious illness.

What are the different forms of depression?

There are several forms of depressive disorders.

Major Depressive Disorder: Major depressive disorder, or major depression, is characterized by a combination of symptoms that interfere with a person's ability to work, sleep, study, eat, and enjoy once-pleasurable activities. Major depression is disabling and prevents a person from functioning normally. Some people may experience only a single episode within their lifetime, but more often a person may have multiple episodes.

Depression is a common but serious illness. Most who experience depression need treatment to get better.

Dysthymic Disorder: Dysthymic disorder, or dysthymia, is characterized by long-term (two years or longer) symptoms that may not be severe enough to disable a person but can prevent normal functioning or feeling well. People with dysthymia may also experience one or more episodes of major depression during their lifetimes.

Minor Depression: Minor depression is characterized by having symptoms for two weeks or longer that do not meet full criteria for major depression. Without treatment, people with minor depression are at high risk for developing major depressive disorder.

Uncharacterized Forms Of Depression: Some forms of depression are slightly different, or they may develop under unique circumstances. However, not everyone agrees on how to characterize and define these forms of depression. They include: psychotic depression, which occurs when a person has severe depression plus some form of psychosis (delusions or hallucinations); postpartum depression, which is much more serious than the "baby blues" that many women experience after giving birth; and seasonal affective disorder (SAD), which is characterized by the onset of depression during the winter months, when there is less natural sunlight. SAD generally lifts during spring and summer and may be effectively treated with light therapy, but nearly half of those with SAD do not get better with light therapy alone. Sufferers may also require psychotherapy in combination with light therapy.

Bipolar Disorder: Bipolar disorder, also called manic-depressive illness, is not as common as major depression or dysthymia. Bipolar disorder is characterized by cycling mood changes—from extreme highs (mania) to extreme lows (depression).

What are the signs and symptoms of depression?

People with depressive illnesses do not all experience the same symptoms. The severity, frequency, and duration of symptoms vary depending on the individual and his or her particular illness.

Signs and symptoms include:

- Persistent sad, anxious, or "empty" feelings
- Feelings of hopelessness or pessimism
- Feelings of guilt, worthlessness, or helplessness
- Irritability or restlessness
- Loss of interest in activities or hobbies once pleasurable
- Fatigue and decreased energy
- Difficulty concentrating, remembering details, and making decisions
- Insomnia, early-morning wakefulness, or excessive sleeping
- Overeating or appetite loss
- Thoughts of suicide or suicide attempts
- Aches or pains, headaches, cramps, or digestive problems that do not ease even with treatment

What causes depression?

Most likely, depression is caused by a combination of genetic, biological, environmental, and psychological factors. Some types of depression tend to run in families. However, depression can occur in people without family histories of depression too. Scientists are studying certain genes that may make some people more prone to depression. In addition, trauma, loss of a loved one, a difficult relationship, or any stressful situation may trigger a depressive episode. Other depressive episodes may occur with or without an obvious trigger.

How do men and women experience depression?

Depression is more common among women than among men. Biological, life cycle, hormonal, and psychosocial factors, that women experience, may be linked to women's higher depression rate. Researchers have shown that hormones directly affect the brain chemistry that controls emotions and mood.

Men often experience depression differently than women. While women with depression are more likely to have feelings of sadness, worthlessness, and excessive guilt, men are more likely to be very tired, irritable, lose interest in once-pleasurable activities, and have difficulty sleeping.

Men may be more likely than women to turn to alcohol or drugs when they are depressed. They also may become frustrated, discouraged, irritable, angry, and sometimes abusive. Some men throw themselves into their work to avoid talking about their depression with family or friends, or behave recklessly. And although more women attempt suicide, many more men die by suicide in the United States.

How do teens experience depression?

Before puberty, boys and girls are equally likely to develop depression. By age 15, however, girls are twice as likely as boys to have had a major depressive episode.

Depression during the teen years comes at a time of great personal change—when boys and girls are forming an identity apart from their parents, grappling with gender issues and emerging sexuality, and making independent decisions for the first time in their lives. Depression in adolescence frequently co-occurs with other disorders such as anxiety, eating disorders, or substance abuse. It can also lead to increased risk for suicide.

How is depression diagnosed and treated?

Depression, even the most severe cases, can be effectively treated. Medications, psychotherapies, and other methods can effectively treat people with depression. The earlier that treatment can begin, the more effective it is.

The first step to getting appropriate treatment is to visit a doctor or mental health specialist. Certain medications, and some medical conditions such as viruses or a thyroid disorder, can cause the same symptoms as depression. A doctor can rule out these possibilities by doing a physical exam, interview, and lab tests. If the doctor can find no medical condition that may be causing the depression, the next step is a psychological evaluation.

The doctor may refer you to a mental health professional, who should discuss with you any family history of depression or other mental disorder and get a complete history of your symptoms. You should discuss when your symptoms started, how long they have lasted, how severe they are, and whether they have occurred before, and, if so, how they were treated. The mental health professional may also ask if you are using alcohol or drugs and if you are thinking about death or suicide.

Once diagnosed, a person with depression can be treated in several ways. The most common treatments are medication and psychotherapy.

How can I help myself if I am depressed?

If you have depression, you may feel exhausted, helpless, and hopeless. It may be extremely difficult to take any action to help yourself, but as you begin to recognize your depression and begin treatment, you will start to feel better. To help yourself, don't wait too long to get evaluated or treated. There is research showing the longer one waits, the greater the impairment can be down the road.

Also, try to be active and exercise and set realistic goals for yourself. Break up large tasks into small ones, set priorities, and do what you can—as you can.

Try to spend time with other people, and confide in a trusted friend or relative. Try not to isolate yourself.

Expect your mood to improve gradually, not immediately. Do not expect to suddenly "snap out of" your depression, so postpone important decisions until you feel better. If you cannot postpone a decision, discuss it with others who know you well and have a more objective view of your situation.

Remember, positive thinking will replace negative thoughts as your depression responds to treatment.

What if I or someone I know is in crisis?

If you are thinking about harming yourself, or know someone who is, tell someone who can help immediately.

- Do not leave your friend or relative alone, if they are in crisis.
- If you are thinking about harming yourself, do not isolate yourself.
- Call your doctor.
- Call 911, or go to a hospital emergency room to get immediate help, or ask a friend or family member to help you do these things.
- Call the toll-free, 24-hour hotline of the National Suicide Prevention Lifeline to talk to a trained counselor:
  - Phone: 1-800-273-TALK (1-800-273-8255)
  - TTY: 1-800-799-4TTY (4889)

Source: National Institute of Mental Health (www.nimh.nih.gov).

Chapter 26

Eating Disorders

What are eating disorders?

An eating disorder is an illness that causes serious disturbances to your everyday diet, such as eating extremely small amounts of food or severely overeating. A person with an eating disorder may have started out just eating smaller or larger amounts of food, but at some point, the urge to eat less or more spiraled out of control. Severe distress or concern about body weight or shape may also characterize an eating disorder.

Eating disorders frequently appear during the teen years or young adulthood but may also develop during childhood or later in life. Common eating disorders include anorexia nervosa, bulimia nervosa, and binge-eating disorder.

Eating disorders affect both men and women. For the latest statistics on eating disorders, see the National Institute of Mental Health (NIMH) website at www.nimh.nih.gov.

It is unknown how many adults and children suffer with other serious, significant eating disorders, including one category of eating disorders called eating disorders not otherwise specified (EDNOS). EDNOS includes eating disorders that do not meet the criteria for anorexia or bulimia nervosa. Binge-eating disorder is a type of eating disorder called EDNOS. EDNOS is the most common diagnosis among people who seek treatment.

Eating disorders are real, treatable medical illnesses. They frequently coexist with other illnesses such as depression, substance abuse, or anxiety disorders. Other symptoms, described in the next section can become life-threatening if a person does not receive treatment. People

About This Chapter: Information for this chapter is excerpted from "Eating Disorders," National Institute of Mental Health (www.nimh.nih.gov), March 2012.

with anorexia nervosa are 18 times more likely to die early compared with people of similar age in the general population.

What are the different types of eating disorders?

Anorexia Nervosa

Anorexia nervosa is characterized by:

- Extreme thinness (emaciation)
- A relentless pursuit of thinness and unwillingness to maintain a normal or healthy weight
- Intense fear of gaining weight
- Distorted body image, a self-esteem that is heavily influenced by perceptions of body weight and shape, or a denial of the seriousness of low body weight
- Lack of menstruation among girls and women
- Extremely restricted eating

Many people with anorexia nervosa see themselves as overweight, even when they are clearly underweight. Eating, food, and weight control become obsessions. People with anorexia nervosa typically weigh themselves repeatedly, portion food carefully, and eat very small quantities of only certain foods. Some people with anorexia nervosa may also engage in binge-eating followed by extreme dieting, excessive exercise, self-induced vomiting, and/or misuse of laxatives, diuretics, or enemas.

Some who have anorexia nervosa recover with treatment after only one episode. Others get well but have relapses. Still others have a more chronic, or long-lasting, form of anorexia nervosa, in which their health declines as they battle the illness.

Other symptoms may develop over time, including:

- Thinning of the bones (osteopenia or osteoporosis)
- Brittle hair and nails
- Dry and yellowish skin
- Growth of fine hair all over the body (lanugo)
- Mild anemia and muscle wasting and weakness
- Severe constipation

- Low blood pressure, slowed breathing, and slowed pulse

- Damage to the structure and function of the heart

- Brain damage

- Multiple organ failure

- Drop in internal body temperature, causing a person to feel cold all the time

- Lethargy, sluggishness, or feeling tired all the time

- Infertility

Bulimia Nervosa

Bulimia nervosa is characterized by recurrent and frequent episodes of eating unusually large amounts of food and feeling a lack of control over these episodes. This binge-eating is followed by behavior that compensates for the overeating such as forced vomiting, excessive use of laxatives or diuretics, fasting, excessive exercise, or a combination of these behaviors.

Unlike anorexia nervosa, people with bulimia nervosa usually maintain what is considered a healthy or normal weight, while some are slightly overweight. But, like people with anorexia nervosa, they often fear gaining weight, want desperately to lose weight, and are intensely unhappy with their body size and shape. Usually, bulimic behavior is done secretly because it is often accompanied by feelings of disgust or shame. The binge-eating and purging cycle happens anywhere from several times a week to many times a day.

Other symptoms include:

- Chronically inflamed and sore throat

- Swollen salivary glands in the neck and jaw area

- Worn tooth enamel, increasingly sensitive and decaying teeth as a result of exposure to stomach acid

- Acid reflux disorder and other gastrointestinal problems

- Intestinal distress and irritation from laxative abuse

- Severe dehydration from purging of fluids

- Electrolyte imbalance (too low or too high levels of sodium, calcium, potassium, and other minerals), which can lead to heart attack

Binge-Eating Disorder

With binge-eating disorder a person loses control over his or her eating. Unlike bulimia nervosa, periods of binge-eating are not followed by purging, excessive exercise, or fasting. As a result, people with binge-eating disorder often are overweight or obese. People with binge-eating disorder who are obese are at higher risk for developing cardiovascular disease and high blood pressure. They also experience guilt, shame, and distress about their binge-eating, which can lead to more binge-eating.

How are eating disorders treated?

Adequate nutrition, reducing excessive exercise, and stopping purging behaviors are the foundations of treatment. Specific forms of psychotherapy, or talk therapy, and medication are effective for many eating disorders. However, in more chronic cases, specific treatments have not yet been identified. Treatment plans often are tailored to individual needs and may include one or more of the following:

- Individual, group, and/or family psychotherapy
- Medical care and monitoring
- Nutritional counseling
- Medications

Some patients may also need to be hospitalized to treat problems caused by malnutrition or to ensure they eat enough if they are very underweight.

Treating Anorexia Nervosa

Treating anorexia nervosa involves three components:

- Restoring the person to a healthy weight
- Treating the psychological issues related to the eating disorder
- Reducing or eliminating behaviors or thoughts that lead to insufficient eating and preventing relapse

Some research suggests that the use of medications, such as antidepressants, antipsychotics, or mood stabilizers, may be modestly effective in treating patients with anorexia nervosa. These medications may help resolve mood and anxiety symptoms that often occur along with anorexia nervosa. It is not clear whether antidepressants can prevent some weight-restored patients with anorexia nervosa from relapsing. Although research is still ongoing, no medication yet has shown to be effective in helping someone gain weight to reach a normal level.

Different forms of psychotherapy, including individual, group, and family-based, can help address the psychological reasons for the illness. In a therapy called the Maudsley approach, parents of adolescents with anorexia nervosa assume responsibility for feeding their child. This approach appears to be very effective in helping people gain weight and improve eating habits and moods. Shown to be effective in case studies and clinical trials, the Maudsley approach is discussed in some guidelines and studies for treating eating disorders in younger, non-chronic patients.

Other research has found that a combined approach of medical attention and supportive psychotherapy, designed specifically for anorexia nervosa patients, is more effective than psychotherapy alone. The effectiveness of a treatment depends on the person involved and his or her situation. Unfortunately, no specific psychotherapy appears to be consistently effective for treating adults with anorexia nervosa. However, research into new treatment and prevention approaches is showing some promise. One study suggests that an online intervention program may prevent some at-risk women from developing an eating disorder. Also, specialized treatment of anorexia nervosa may help reduce the risk of death.

Treating Bulimia Nervosa

As with anorexia nervosa, treatment for bulimia nervosa often involves a combination of options and depends upon the needs of the individual. To reduce or eliminate binge-eating and purging behaviors, a patient may undergo nutritional counseling and psychotherapy, especially cognitive behavioral therapy (CBT), or be prescribed medication. CBT helps a person focus on his or her current problems and how to solve them. The therapist helps the patient learn how to identify distorted or unhelpful thinking patterns, recognize and change inaccurate beliefs, relate to others in more positive ways, and change behaviors accordingly.

CBT that is tailored to treat bulimia nervosa is effective in changing binge-eating and purging behaviors and eating attitudes. Therapy may be individual or group-based.

Some antidepressants, such as fluoxetine (Prozac), which is the only medication approved by the U.S. Food and Drug Administration (FDA) for treating bulimia nervosa, may help patients who also have depression or anxiety. Fluoxetine also appears to help reduce binge-eating and purging behaviors, reduce the chance of relapse, and improve eating attitudes.

Treating Binge-Eating Disorder

Treatment options for binge-eating disorder are similar to those used to treat bulimia nervosa. Psychotherapy, especially CBT that is tailored to the individual, has been shown to be effective. Again, this type of therapy can be offered in an individual or group environment.

Fluoxetine and other antidepressants may reduce binge-eating episodes and help lessen depression in some patients.

How are males affected?

Like females who have eating disorders, males also have a distorted sense of body image. For some, their symptoms are similar to those seen in females. Others may have muscle dysmorphia, a type of disorder that is characterized by an extreme concern with becoming more muscular. Unlike girls with eating disorders, who mostly want to lose weight, some boys with muscle dysmorphia see themselves as smaller than they really are and want to gain weight or bulk up. Men and boys are more likely to use steroids or other dangerous drugs to increase muscle mass.

Although males with eating disorders exhibit the same signs and symptoms as females, they are less likely to be diagnosed with what is often considered a female disorder. More research is needed to understand the unique features of these disorders among males.

What is being done to better understand and treat eating disorders?

Researchers are finding that eating disorders are caused by a complex interaction of genetic, biological, behavioral, psychological, and social factors. But many questions still need answers. Researchers are using the latest in technology and science to better understand eating disorders.

One approach involves the study of human genes. Researchers are studying various combinations of genes to determine if any deoxyribonucleic acid (DNA) variations are linked to the risk of developing eating disorders.

FDA Warnings On Antidepressants

Antidepressants are safe and popular, but some studies have suggested that they may have unintentional effects on some people, especially in adolescents and young adults. The FDA warning says that patients of all ages taking antidepressants should be watched closely, especially during the first few weeks of treatment. Possible side effects to look for are depression that gets worse, suicidal thinking or behavior, or any unusual changes in behavior such as trouble sleeping, agitation, or withdrawal from normal social situations. Families and caregivers should report any changes to the doctor.

Neuroimaging studies are also providing a better understanding of eating disorders and possible treatments. One study showed different patterns of brain activity between women with bulimia nervosa and healthy women. Using functional magnetic resonance imaging (fMRI), researchers were able to see the differences in brain activity while the women performed a task that involved self-regulation (a task that requires overcoming an automatic or impulsive response).

Psychotherapy interventions are also being studied. One such study of adolescents found that more adolescents with bulimia nervosa recovered after receiving Maudsley model family-based treatment than those receiving supportive psychotherapy that did not specifically address the eating disorder.

Researchers are studying questions about behavior, genetics, and brain function to better understand risk factors, identify biological markers, and develop specific psychotherapies and medications that can target areas in the brain that control eating behavior. Neuroimaging and genetic studies may provide clues for how each person may respond to specific treatments for these medical illnesses.

Chapter 27

Body Dysmorphic Disorder

Body dysmorphic disorder (BDD) is a mental illness. People who have this illness constantly worry about the way they look. They may think something that isn't there, or that others don't even notice, is a serious defect. The severity of BDD varies. For example, some people know their feelings aren't rational or justified, while others are almost delusional in their conviction.

BDD causes severe emotional distress. It is not just vanity and is not something a person can just "forget about" or "get over." The preoccupation can be so extreme that the affected person has trouble functioning at work, school, or in social situations. Any part of the body can be targeted.

It is thought that between one and two per cent of the population may have BDD, with men and women equally affected. BDD usually starts in the teenage years, when concern over physical appearance is common. Suicide rates among people with BDD are high. If you suspect you have BDD, see your doctor or a mental health professional.

Common Areas Of Concern

Common areas of concern include:

- Facial skin

- Face, including the size or shape of the eyes, nose, ears, and lips

- Size or shape of virtually any body part including buttocks, thighs, abdomen, legs, breasts, and genitals

About This Chapter: Information in this chapter is reprinted from "Body Dysmorphic Disorder," Better Health Channel, www.betterhealth.vic.gov.au. © 2013State Government of Victoria. All rights reserved.

- Overall size and shape of the body
- Symmetry of the body or particular body parts

Symptoms

Symptoms can vary according to which body part (or parts) is targeted, but general symptoms of BDD include:

- Thinking about the perceived defect for hours every day
- Worrying about their failure to match the "physical perfection" of models and celebrities
- Distress about their preoccupation
- Constantly asking trusted loved ones for reassurance about their looks, but not believing the answer
- Constantly looking at their reflection or taking pains to avoid catching their reflection (for example, throwing away or covering up mirrors)
- Constant dieting and over exercising
- Grooming to excess—for example, shaving the same patch of skin over and over
- Avoiding any situation they feel will call attention to their defect. In extreme cases, this can mean never leaving home
- Taking great pains to hide or camouflage the "defect"
- Squeezing or picking at skin blemishes for hours on end
- Wanting dermatological treatment or cosmetic surgery, even when professionals believe the treatment is unnecessary
- Repeat cosmetic surgery procedures, especially if the same body part is being "improved" with each procedure
- Depression and anxiety, including suicidal thoughts

The Cause Is Unknown

The cause of BDD is unknown. Theories include:

- A person with BDD has a genetic tendency to develop this type of mental illness. The trigger may be the stress of adolescence.

- Particular drugs, such as ecstasy, may trigger onset in susceptible people.

- BDD could be caused by chemical imbalances in the brain.

- A person with low self-esteem who has impossible standards of perfection judges some part of their body as ugly. Over time, this behaviour becomes more and more compulsive.

- Western society's narrow standards of beauty may trigger BDD in vulnerable people.

Similarities To Other Conditions

BDD is similar to other conditions, including:

- **Agoraphobia:** A type of anxiety disorder characterised by the fear of situations or places from which escape seems difficult [is agoraphobia]. In extreme cases, a person with agoraphobia is housebound. However, a person who stays home out of fear of publicly exposing their defect may have BDD instead of agoraphobia.

- **Anorexia Nervosa:** BDD is often misdiagnosed as anorexia nervosa because of the preoccupation with appearance. However, anorexia nervosa is characterised by the drive to control one's weight. It's possible for a person to have anorexia nervosa and BDD at the same time.

- **Hypochondriasis:** The preoccupation with the development of disease [is hypochondriasis]. However, the person with BDD is preoccupied with their looks, not their health.

- **Obsessive Compulsive Disorder (OCD):** [OCD is] characterised by recurring unwanted thoughts and images (obsessions) and repetitive rituals (compulsions). As people with BDD are obsessively preoccupied with an aspect of their appearance, it has been proposed that BDD may be a form of OCD. In addition, some people diagnosed with BDD have or have had OCD.

- **Social Phobia:** A type of anxiety disorder, characterised by fear of interaction with people. A person with social phobia may worry about being judged, criticised, ridiculed or humiliated. If the avoidance is triggered by concerns about their appearance, the underlying problem may be BDD.

- **Trichotillomania:** The irresistible urge to pluck or pull out hairs. If the behaviour is triggered by concerns about appearance, the underlying problem may be BDD. Picking or squeezing at skin blemishes for hours at a time is a similar condition to trichotillomania.

Diagnosis Is Difficult

Diagnosis of BDD is difficult for many reasons, including:

- The person with BDD is more likely to seek help from dermatologists and cosmetic surgeons rather than psychologists and psychiatrists.

- The person with BDD is ashamed and doesn't want to seek help from mental health professionals.

- This type of mental illness doesn't get much publicity, so some health professionals may not even be aware that BDD exists.

- BDD is similar to many other conditions and misdiagnosis is possible

Treatment

There has been little research into the effectiveness of treatment for BDD. However, treatment that seems to help the most includes a combination of:

- **Cognitive Behaviour Therapy (CBT):** training in how to change underlying attitudes in order to think and feel in different ways. This includes learning to tolerate the distress of "exposing" their perceived defect to others.

- **Coping And Management Skills:** training in how to cope with symptoms of anxiety. For example, the person may learn relaxation techniques and how to combat hyperventilation.

- **Drugs:** including antidepressant medications, particularly selective serotonin reuptake inhibitors (SSRIs). These drugs help reduce many BDD symptoms, including the compulsive thoughts, depression and anxiety. Generally, drugs are used in combination with psychotherapy.

Things To Remember

- Body dysmorphic disorder (BDD) is a mental illness characterised by the constant worrying over a perceived or slight defect in appearance.
- BDD usually starts in the teenage years, when concern over physical appearance is common.
- Treatment includes cognitive behaviour therapy and antidepressant drugs.
- If you suspect you have BDD, see your doctor or mental health professional.

Some people with body dysmorphic disorder seek cosmetic surgery to "correct" an actual or perceived physical flaw. Medical experts are divided on the ethics of what is sometimes called "non-therapeutic mutilation" or extreme body modification. Any medical or surgical procedure carries health risks. Unnecessary attempts to change one's appearance through surgery may lead to dissatisfaction with the results and could worsen a person's BBD.

Where To Get Help

- Your doctor

- Local community mental health centre

- Psychologist

- Psychiatrist

Chapter 28

Self-Injury

What does hurting yourself mean?

Hurting yourself, sometimes called self-injury, is when a person deliberately hurts his or her own body. Some self-injuries can leave scars that won't go away, while others leave marks or bruises that eventually will go away. These are some forms of self-injury:

- Cutting yourself (such as using a razor blade, knife, or other sharp object to cut the skin)
- Punching yourself or punching things (like a wall)
- Burning yourself with cigarettes, matches, or candles
- Pulling out your hair
- Poking objects through body openings
- Breaking your bones or bruising yourself

Why do some teens want to hurt themselves?

Many people cut themselves because it gives them a sense of relief. Some people use cutting as a means to cope with a problem. Some teens say that when they hurt themselves, they are trying to stop feeling lonely, angry, or hopeless. Some teens who hurt themselves have low self-esteem, they may feel unloved by their family and friends, and they may have an eating disorder, an alcohol or drug problem, or may have been victims of abuse.

Teens who hurt themselves often keep their feelings "bottled up" inside and have a hard time letting their feelings show. Some teens who hurt themselves say that feeling the pain provides a sense of relief from intense feelings. Cutting can relieve the tension from bottled up sadness or

About This Chapter: Information in this chapter are from "Cutting and Hurting Yourself: Your Feelings," Office on Women's Health (www.girlshealth.gov), May 2010.

anxiety. Others hurt themselves in order to "feel." Often people who hold back strong emotions can begin feeling numb and cutting can be a way to cope with this because it causes them to feel something. Some teens also may hurt themselves because they want to fit in with others who do it.

Self-Harm And Trauma

What is self-harm?

Self-harm refers to a person's harming their own body on purpose. Other terms for self-harm are "self-abuse" or "cutting." Overall, a person who self-harms does not mean to kill him or herself.

Self-harm tends to begin in teen or early adult years. Some people may engage in self-harm a few times and then stop. Others engage in it more often and have trouble stopping the behavior. Self-harm is related to trauma in that those who self-harm are likely to have been abused in childhood.

How common is self-harm?

The rates of self-harm vary widely, depending on how researchers pose their questions about it. It is estimated that in the general public, 2–6% engage in self-harm at some point in their lives. Among students, the rates are higher, ranging from 13–35%.

Rates of self-harm are also higher among those in treatment for mental health problems. Those in treatment who have a diagnosis of posttraumatic stress disorder (PTSD) are more likely to engage in self-harm than those without PTSD.

What are self-harmers like?

Self-harmers, as compared to others, have more frequent and more negative feelings such as fear or worry, depression, and aggressive impulses. Links have also been found between self-harm and feeling numb or feeling as if you're outside your body. Often those who self-harm have low self-esteem, and they do not tend to express their feelings.

Those who self-harm appear to have higher rates of PTSD and other mental health problems. Self-harm is most often related to going through trauma in childhood rather than as an adult. Those who self-harm have high rates of:

- Childhood sexual abuse
- Childhood physical abuse
- Emotional neglect
- Bonds with caregivers that are not stable or secure
- Long separations from caregivers

If you are hurting yourself, **please get help**—it is possible to overcome the urge to cut. There are other ways to find relief and cope with your emotions. Please talk to your parents, your doctor, or an adult you trust, like a teacher or religious leader.

Those who self-harm very often have a history of childhood sexual abuse. For example, in one group of self-harmers, 93% said they had been sexually abused in childhood. Some research has looked at whether certain aspects of childhood sexual abuse increase the risk that survivors will engage in self-harm as adults. The findings show that more severe, more frequent, or longer-lasting sexual abuse is linked to an increased risk of engaging in self-harm in one's adult years.

Why do people engage in self-harm?

While many ideas have been offered, the answer to this question may vary from person to person. Research on the reasons for self-harm suggests that people engage in self-harm to:

- Decrease symptoms of feeling numb or as if you are outside your body or yourself
- Reduce stress and tension
- Block upsetting memories and flashbacks
- Show a need for help
- Ensure safety and protection
- Express and release distress
- Reduce anger
- Punish self
- Hurt self instead of others

How is self-harm treated?

Self-harm is a problem that many people are embarrassed or ashamed to discuss. Often, they try to hide their self-harm behaviors. They may hold back from getting mental health or even medical treatment.

Self-harm is often seen with other mental health problems like PTSD or substance abuse. For this reason, it does not tend to be treated separately from the other mental health problems. Some research suggests, though, that adding in a round of therapy focused just on the self-harming behavior may result in less self-harming.

There have not yet been strong studies on using medicine to treat self-harm behaviors. For this reason, experts have not reached agreement on whether medicines should be used to treat self-harm behaviors.

Source: Information in this box is excerpted from "Self-Harm and Trauma," United States Department of Veterans Affairs, National Center for Posttraumatic Stress Disorder (PTSD) (www.ptsd.va.gov), December 2011.

Who are the people who hurt themselves?

People who hurt themselves come from all walks of life, no matter their age, gender, race, or ethnicity. About one in 100 people hurts himself or herself on purpose. More females hurt themselves than males. Teens usually hurt themselves by cutting with sharp objects.

What are the signs of self-injury?

These are some signs of self-injury:

- Cuts or scars on the arms or legs that you can see

- Hiding cuts or scars by wearing long-sleeved shirts or pants, even in hot weather

- Making poor excuses about how the injuries happened

Self-injury can be dangerous. Cutting can lead to infections, scars, numbness, and even hospitalization or death. People who share tools to cut themselves are at risk of getting and spreading diseases like HIV and hepatitis. Teens who continue to hurt themselves are less likely to learn how to cope with negative feelings.

Are you or a friend depressed, angry, or having a hard time coping with life?

If you are thinking about hurting yourself, **please ask for help**! Talk with an adult you trust, like a teacher, minister, or doctor. There is nothing wrong with asking for help. Everyone needs help sometimes. You have a right to be strong, safe, and happy!

Do you have a friend who hurts herself or himself?

Please try to get your friend to talk to a trusted adult. Your friend may need professional counseling and treatment. Help is available. Counselors can teach positive ways to cope with problems without turning to self-injury. If your friend won't talk to a trusted adult, you should tell an adult you trust about the situation.

Have you been pressured to cut yourself by others who do it?

If so, think about how much you value that friendship or relationship. Do you really want a friend who wants you to hurt yourself, wants to cause you pain, and/or wants to put you in danger? Try to hang out with other friends who don't pressure you in this way.

Chapter 29

Loss And Grief

Grief is the term used to describe the feelings we have after a loss. It is natural to feel overwhelmed with emotions like pain, anger, and sadness. Sometimes you can even feel numb.

This chapter is about dealing with the grief after the loss of someone or something really important to you. It looks at doing things in your own style, your own time and in a healthy way.

Loss

Loss can come into our lives in lots of ways, and it affects each of us differently. One of the biggest and most difficult losses is the death of someone really important to you.

There are many types of loss where you might experience sadness, confusion, and anger.

- The death of someone you love

- The death of a pet

- Your parents or other important people splitting up or getting divorced

- Separation from a parent, both parents, or your family

- Separation from friends or your community

- Moving away from home or leaving your country

- Splitting up with your partner

About This Chapter: Reprinted with permission from Women's and Children's Health Network (www.cyh.com) © 2011Government of South Australia.

- Being forced to give up something you want to keep (like your job, your child, or your home)

- Losing your job

- Leaving school or university

- Losing the ability to do some things through disability

- Becoming really sick or seeing someone else become really sick

Even when something happens that appears positive, such as leaving school and starting work, we can experience some feelings of grief for what we've left behind.

When we have a loss in our life, we go through reactions of grief. These reactions and feelings are different for everyone. You always feel loss in your own unique way.

What Is Grief?

When you grieve you might notice some of these feelings. You might not feel all of them, and you might not feel them in the same order.

- **Denial, Shock, Or Disbelief:** This is like a temporary relief and helps you to avoid getting completely taken over by grief ("It hasn't really happened," "This isn't real," "I must be dreaming," "She is just fooling around," or "He will be back.").

- **Questions, Questions, Questions:** You try to make sense of the loss. These might be related to feelings of guilt ("Why didn't I?" "If only I had …," or "I should have …") or [feelings of] confusion ("What is going on?" "I don't understand," or "What happened?").

- **Anxiety:** Loss can be scary. You might think about your future ("What will I do?" or "How will I cope?") or have a fear of losing control ("I'm going to lose it," "I can't stop it," or "What else might I lose without me being able to stop it?").

- **Anger:** Anger comes from other feelings, like feeling abandoned, hurt, or scared. You might express anger in lots of ways. You might direct your anger at people you think caused the loss ("Why did you?" "You always …," or "You never cared.") or feel helplessness ("I couldn't stop it," "I can't change anything," or "I can't cope.").

- **Crying, Sobbing, Depression:** Sadness might feel like a black cloud over your whole world. You might long for what you have lost. You might lose interest in life— you don't want to go out, or see, or do things you usually do. You might feel loneliness, or feel you have no one to turn to.

- **Reality And Acceptance (and adjusting to new life patterns):** You realize what has happened and the pain does not hurt so much. Everything is different but the struggle is not so huge. Life goes on with the memories and experience of knowing what you once had. You start looking toward the future.

- **Grief:** [Grief] can cause physical symptoms like headaches, feeling sick in the stomach, aching muscles, feeling run down, trouble sleeping, feeling tired, [and/or] having no energy. You might find you get sick more easily.

These feelings can happen at any time and for any length of time. You might have more than one at once. You might feel really good one day and awful the next. Special times like Christmas, birthdays, or anniversaries can be difficult. You may return to a feeling and go through it again. Sometimes it can feel worse in the morning or as you are about to go to sleep. Sometimes you might wonder if you will ever feel "normal" again. You will—gradually the pain is with you less often, and life finds a new sense of meaning.

If you find you are stuck in one of these feelings, and not gradually "moving on" over time, it would be a good idea to talk to a counselor about it.

Dealing With Loss In Harmful Ways

Grief affects you in lots of ways. Not only do you have a rush of emotions that can be hard to cope with, but you might also do things that can be harmful.

- **You might use drugs and alcohol,** [trying] and cover up the pain or make it go away. Many people think using drugs or alcohol is the only way (or a good way) to deal with the pain, but this method may just "put off" or prolong the natural process of grief, as well as doing you harm.

- **You might hurt other people.** It's natural to feel angry when you grieve. Anger is sometimes the emotion you show when there are a whole heap of other emotions happening underneath. If you think you've no safe place to express yourself, or don't understand what's going on, you might turn anger on other people. Anger is a natural emotion; violence is a chosen behavior. Anger can be expressed in a safe way without hurting others.

- **You might hurt yourself.** Choosing to hurt yourself is only one choice to express the pain that is happening for you. There are lots of other ways you can choose to express yourself.

If you have chosen any of these things, it can be useful to talk to someone you trust or find other ways to express yourself. Some people express themselves through art or music; others like to write down what they are feeling. This can also be a stepping stone to explaining how you feel to other people.

Tips To Help

- **Accept your own feelings.** Understand that what you are feeling is natural. Let yourself cry, talk about the loss, or have a laugh. Check out the stages of grief. Let yourself feel what you are feeling. The feeling will pass.

- **Express your feelings.** Talk to someone you trust. Write a letter, poetry, or a journal. Paint, draw, or sing. Express what you are feeling—your fear, your hurt, and your loss. Talk about what you have gained by knowing the person or having the experience you have had. Talk about the good and not-so-good times.

- **[Go to] ceremonies.** Funerals, ceremonies, or memorials can be important. They are opportunities to share your grief with other people or help accept the end of a part of your life. This is an ending of one phase in your life and the beginning of a new one. Maybe you could do something special with friends and family, like have a remembrance meal.

- **Take each step at a time.** Live each day as it comes. Understand and accept disruption in your life. Take control of things you can. Understand there are things you have little or no control over. Give yourself permission to grieve.

- **Move forward.** What have you learned from that person, place, or experience? What memories do you have? How have they become part of your life? How might you carry these [memories] on? How might you share them with children or others? What place might these skills, attributes, stories, or knowledge hold in your future?

- **[Find a] support.** Support is essential. Talk to a friend, family, or someone you trust. Sometimes it might feel people "don't understand" or "get sick of your grieving." It can be useful to [talk to] a counselor or have a network of supports in your life.

- **Have a laugh.** Your sense of humor can be a great tool at any hard time. It is OK to laugh at things you would usually laugh at. Advantages of laughter are that they give you just a little break from the pain and release healthy, healing chemicals into your body.

- **Celebrate your memory.** Plant something as a living memorial. Carry or wear something that reminds you of the person who died or the thing you have lost. Create a memory book or journal with photos, stories, pictures, or poems. Put up a photo or something else that reminds you of that person. Spend time at a place or doing things that you used to do.

- **Explore your spirituality.** Pray, meditate, or spend some time with nature. Use your own personal spirituality to explore what death or loss means to you and your spiritual self.

- **Change.** Be open to new ways of doing things. When it feels right, start something new. Don't feel guilty about this. It is part of healing, and you will never lose what your relationship with the person you have lost has given you.

- **Be aware.** It is natural to become more dependent on others immediately after a loss. It is not useful to keep this going for a long time. Keep an eye out for signs that indicate that you are not gradually feeling better. Give yourself a pat on the back when you do things for yourself.

- **Reward yourself.** Be kind to yourself. Do things you like doing. Treat yourself to things that make you happy. When you feel ready, do something to help someone else. Soak up the enjoyment as much as you can!

- **Write down the things you have learned.** What have you noticed about yourself in this time? What have you found hardest? How did you overcome the hard things? What did you find easiest? What does this tell you about yourself? What have you learned about your life? What beliefs have you gained, let go of, or are new to you? How might you use this knowledge in your future? If you write it down, you will see how you are gradually feeling better.

Note: It is not usually a good idea to make major life changing decisions in the first few months after the loss. It is often better to wait until your life is back in balance again.

Remember that others around you may be feeling grief too. You may be able to help them.

Does Grief Affect People Differently?

Sure does! Some people don't like to make a fuss; others let everyone know how they are feeling. Men and women are treated differently in our society. This can mean they may express their grief differently. Different cultures and religions see death, loss, and grief in different ways. How you express your grief—and the meaning you give to loss—will be in your own way, based on your own beliefs and view of the world.

When you are grieving for someone or something you have lost, it is natural to feel that you are alone in this. Everyone in the world has to deal with loss. Know that you are not alone, and reach out to others. Some may not be good at supporting you, but all will understand what you are going through.

Chapter 30

Dealing With Depression

The teenage years can be tough, and it's perfectly normal to feel sad or irritable every now and then. But if these feelings don't go away or become so intense that you can't handle them, you may be suffering from depression. The good news is that you don't have to feel this way. Help is available and you have more power than you think. There are many things you can do to help yourself or a friend start feeling better.

What Depression Feels Like

When you're depressed, it can feel like no one understands. But depression is far more common in teens than you may think. You are not alone and your depression is not a hopeless case. Even though it can feel like depression will never lift, it eventually will—and with proper treatment and healthy choices, that day can come even sooner.

Signs And Symptoms Of Teen Depression

It's hard to put into words how depression feels, and people experience it differently. There are, however, some common problems and symptoms that teens with depression experience.

- You constantly feel irritable, sad, or angry.
- Nothing seems fun anymore, and you just don't see the point of trying.
- You feel bad about yourself—worthless, guilty, or just "wrong" in some way.
- You sleep too much or not enough.

About This Chapter: "Teen Depression: Guide for Teenagers" by Suzanne Barston, Melinda Smith, MA, and Jeanne Segal, PhD, updated January 2013. © 2013 Helpguide.org. All rights reserved. Helpguide provides a detailed list of references and resources for this article, with links to related Helpguide topics and information from other websites. For a complete list of these resources, go to http://www.helpguide.org/mental/depression_teen_teenagers.htm.

- You have frequent, unexplained headaches or other physical problems.

- Anything and everything makes you cry.

- You've gained or lost weight without consciously trying to.

- You just can't concentrate. Your grades may be plummeting because of it.

- You feel helpless and hopeless.

- You're thinking about death or suicide. (If this is true, talk to someone right away!)

When Teen Depression Turns Deadly

If your feelings become so overwhelming that you can't see any solution besides harming yourself or others, you need to get help right away. And yet, asking for help when you're in the midst of such strong emotions can be really tough. If talking to a stranger might be easier for you, call 1-800-273-TALK in the U.S. to speak in confidence to someone who can understand and help you deal with your feelings. To find a suicide helpline outside the U.S., visit Befrienders Worldwide at www.befrienders.org.

Is Your Friend Depressed?

If you're a teenager with a friend who seems down or troubled, you may suspect depression. But how do you know it's not just a passing phase or a bad mood? Look for common warning signs of teen depression:

- Your friend doesn't want to do the things you guys used to love to do.
- Your friend starts using alcohol or drugs or hanging with a bad crowd.
- Your friend stops going to classes and afterschool activities.
- Your friend talks about being bad, ugly, stupid, or worthless.
- Your friend starts talking about death or suicide.

Coping With Suicidal Thoughts

In the meantime, the following suggestions can help get you through until you feel ready to talk to someone:

- There is ALWAYS another solution, even if you can't see it right now. Many kids who have attempted suicide (and survived) say that they did it because they mistakenly felt there was no other solution to a problem they were experiencing. At the time, they could not see another way out, but in truth, they didn't really want to die. Remember that, no matter how horribly you feel, these emotions will pass.

- Having thoughts of hurting yourself or others does not make you a bad person. Depression can make you think and feel things that are out of character. No one should judge you or condemn you for these feelings if you are brave enough to talk about them.

- If your feelings are uncontrollable, tell yourself to wait 24 hours before you take any action. This can give you time to really think things through and give yourself some distance from the strong emotions that are plaguing you. During this 24-hour period, try to talk to someone—anyone—as long as they are not another suicidal or depressed person. Call a hotline or talk to a friend. What do you have to lose?

- If you're afraid you can't control yourself, make sure you are never alone. Even if you can't verbalize your feelings, just stay in public places, hang out with friends or family members, or go to a movie—anything to keep from being by yourself and in danger.

Above all, do not do anything that could result in permanent damage or death to yourself or others. Remember, suicide is a "permanent solution to a temporary problem." Help is available. All you need to do is take that first step and reach out.

Talking To An Adult You Trust About Teen Depression

As Will Smith once said, "parents just don't understand." Understatement of the year, huh? It may seem like there's no way your parents will be able to help, especially if they are always nagging you or getting angry about your behavior. The truth is, parents hate to see their kids hurting. They may feel frustrated because they don't understand what is going on with you or know how to help.

Many parents don't know enough about depression to recognize it in their own kids. So, it may be up to you to educate them. You can refer them to this chapter, or look for further information online. Letting your parents know that you are feeling depressed will probably motivate them to get you the help you need.

If your parents are abusive in any way, or if they have problems of their own that makes it difficult for them to take care of you, find another adult you trust (such as a relative, teacher, counselor, or coach). This person can either help you approach your parents or direct you toward the support you need. If you truly don't have anyone you can talk to, there are many hotlines, services, and support groups that can help.

No matter what, talk to someone, especially if you are having any thoughts of harming yourself or others. Asking for help is the bravest thing you can do, and the first step on your way to feeling better.

The Importance Of Accepting And Sharing Your Feelings

It can be hard to open up about how you're feeling—especially when you're feeling depressed, hopeless, ashamed, or worthless.

It's important to remember that everyone struggles with feelings like these at one time or another. They don't mean you're weak, fundamentally flawed, or no good. Accepting your feelings and opening up about them with someone you trust will help you feel less alone.

No matter what it feels like, people love and care about you, and if you can muster the courage to talk about your depression, it can—and will—be resolved. Some people think that talking about sad feelings will make them worse, but the opposite is almost always true. It is very helpful to share your worries with someone who will listen and care.

What You Can Do To Feel Better: Tips For Depressed Teens

Depression is not your fault, and you didn't do anything to cause it. However, you do have some control over feeling better. Staying connected to friends and family, making healthy lifestyle decisions, and keeping stress under control can all have a hugely positive impact on your mood.

In the meantime, you might need therapy or medication to help you while you sort out your feelings. Look into your treatment options with your parents. If medication is being considered, do your research before making a decision, as some antidepressants used for adults can actually make teens feel worse.

Try Not To Isolate Yourself

When you're depressed, you may not feel like seeing anybody or doing anything. Just getting out of bed in the morning can be difficult, but isolating yourself only makes depression worse. Make it a point to stay social—even if that's the last thing you want to do. As you get out into the world, you may find yourself feeling better.

Beating Depression, One Day At A Time

You can't beat depression through sheer willpower, but you do have some control—even if your depression is severe and stubbornly persistent. The key to depression recovery is to start with a few small goals and slowly build from there.

Spend time with friends, especially those who are active, upbeat, and make you feel good about yourself. Avoid hanging out with those who abuse drugs or alcohol, get you into trouble, or who make you feel insecure. It's also a good idea to limit the time you spend playing video games or surfing online.

Keep Your Body Healthy

Making healthy lifestyle choices can do wonders for your mood. Things like diet and exercise have been shown to help depression. Ever heard of a "runners high?" You actually get a rush of endorphins from exercising, which makes you feel instantly happier. Physical activity can be as effective as medications or therapy for depression, so get involved in sports, ride your bike, or take a dance class. Any activity helps! Even a short walk can be beneficial.

As for food, it's true that you are what you eat. An improper diet can make you feel sluggish and tired, which worsens depression symptoms. Your body needs vitamins and minerals such as iron and the B-vitamins. Make sure you're feeding your mind with plenty of fruits, vegetables, and whole grains. Talk to your parents, doctor, or school nurse about how to ensure your diet is adequately nutritious.

Avoid Alcohol And Drugs

You may be tempted to drink or use drugs in an effort to escape from your feelings and get a "mood boost," even if just for a short time. However, substance use can not only make depression worse, but can cause you to become depressed in the first place. Alcohol and drug use can also increase suicidal feelings. In short, drinking and taking drugs will make you feel worse—not better—in the long run.

If you're addicted to alcohol or drugs, seek help. You will need special treatment for your substance problem on top of whatever treatment you're receiving for your depression.

Ask For Help If You're Stressed

Stress and worry can take a big toll, even leading to depression. Talk to a teacher or school counselor if exams or classes seem overwhelming. Likewise, if you have a health concern you feel you can't talk to your parents about—such as a pregnancy scare or drug problem—seek medical attention at a clinic or see a doctor. A health professional can help you approach your parents (if that is required) and guide you toward appropriate treatment.

If you're dealing with relationship, friendship, or family problems, talk to an adult you trust. Your school may have a counselor you can go to for help, or you may want to ask your parents to make an appointment for you to see a therapist.

Helping A Depressed Friend

Depressed teens typically rely on their friends more than their parents or other adults in their lives, so you may find yourself in the position of being the first—or only—person that they talk to about their feelings. While this might seem like a huge responsibility, there are many things you can do to help.

- **Get your friend to talk to you.** Starting a conversation about depression can be daunting, but you can say something simple: "You seem like you are really down, and not yourself. I really want to help you. Is there anything I can do?"

- **Know that your friend doesn't expect you to have the answers.** Your friend probably just needs someone to listen and be supportive. By listening and responding in a non-judgmental and reassuring manner, you are helping in a major way.

- **Encourage your friend to get help.** Urge your depressed friend to talk to a parent, teacher, or counselor. It might be scary for your friend to admit to an authority figure that there is a problem. Having you there might help, so offer to go along for support.

- **Stick with your friend through the hard times.** Depression can make people do and say things that are hurtful or strange. But your friend is going through a very difficult time, so try not to take it personally. Once your friend gets help, he or she will go back to being the person you know and love. In the meantime, make sure you have other friends or family taking care of you. Your feelings are important and need to be respected, too.

- **Speak up if your friend is suicidal.** If your friend is joking or talking about suicide, giving possessions away, or saying goodbye, tell a trusted adult immediately. Your only responsibility at this point is to get your friend help, and get it fast. Even if you promised not to tell, your friend needs your help. It's better to have a friend who is temporarily angry at you than one who is no longer alive.

If You Are Suffering And Don't Know Where To Turn...

- In the U.S., call the Nineline.org hotline for children and teens at 1-800-999-9999. It's free, confidential, and available from 4:00 PM to 8:00 PM, Eastern Time, seven days a week.
- In the UK, call the Childline.org.uk helpline for children and teens at 0800 1111.
- In Australia, call the Lifeline.org.aus 24-hour helpline at 13 11 14.
- In Canada, call the KidsHelpPhone.ca helpline at 1-800-668-6868.

Chapter 31

Suicide

[**Ed. Note:** Although some of the text in this chapter addresses parents, teens will still find the information pertinent.]

The tragedy of a young person dying because of overwhelming hopelessness or frustration is devastating to family, friends, and community. Parents, siblings, classmates, coaches, and neighbors might be left wondering if they could have done something to prevent that young person from turning to suicide.

Learning more about factors that might lead an adolescent to suicide may help prevent further tragedies. Even though it's not always preventable, it's always a good idea to be informed and take action to help a troubled teenager.

About Teen Suicide

The reasons behind a teen's suicide or attempted suicide can be complex. Although suicide is relatively rare among children, the rate of suicides and suicide attempts increases tremendously during adolescence.

Suicide is the third-leading cause of death for 15- to 24-year-olds, according to the Centers for Disease Control and Prevention (CDC), after accidents and homicide. It's also thought that at least 25 attempts are made for every completed teen suicide.

About This Chapter: "About Teen Suicide," January 2011, is reprinted with permission from www.kidshealth .org. This information was provided by KidsHealth®, one of the largest resources online for medically reviewed health information written for parents, kids, and teens. For more articles like this, visit www.KidsHealth.org, or www.TeensHealth.org. Copyright © 1995–2012 The Nemours Foundation. All rights reserved.

The risk of suicide increases dramatically when kids and teens have access to firearms at home, and nearly 60% of all suicides in the United States are committed with a gun. That's why any gun in your home should be unloaded, locked, and kept out of the reach of children and teens.

Overdose using over-the-counter, prescription, and non-prescription medicine is also a very common method for both attempting and completing suicide. It's important to monitor carefully all medications in your home. Also be aware that teens will "trade" different prescription medications at school and carry them (or store them) in their locker or backpack.

Suicide rates differ between boys and girls. Girls think about and attempt suicide about twice as often as boys, and tend to attempt suicide by overdosing on drugs or cutting themselves. Yet boys die by suicide about four times as often girls, perhaps because they tend to use more lethal methods, such as firearms, hanging, or jumping from heights.

Which Teens Are At Risk For Suicide?

It can be hard to remember how it felt to be a teen, caught in that gray area between childhood and adulthood. Sure, it's a time of tremendous possibility but it also can be a period of stress and worry. There's pressure to fit in socially, to perform academically, and to act responsibly.

Adolescence is also a time of sexual identity and relationships and a need for independence that often conflicts with the rules and expectations set by others.

Young people with mental health problems—such as anxiety, depression, bipolar disorder, or insomnia—are at higher risk for suicidal thoughts. Teens going through major life changes (parents' divorce, moving, a parent leaving home due to military service or parental separation, financial changes) and those who are victims of bullying are at greater risk of suicidal thoughts.

Factors that increase the risk of suicide among teens include:

- A psychological disorder, especially depression, bipolar disorder, and alcohol and drug use (in fact, approximately 95% of people who die by suicide have a psychological disorder at the time of death)

- Feelings of distress, irritability, or agitation

- Feelings of hopelessness and worthlessness that often accompany depression

- A previous suicide attempt

- A family history of depression or suicide

- Emotional, physical, or sexual abuse

- Lack of a support network, poor relationships with parents or peers, and feelings of social isolation
- Dealing with bisexuality or homosexuality in an unsupportive family or community or hostile school environment

Warning Signs

Suicide among teens often occurs following a stressful life event, such as problems at school, a breakup with a boyfriend or girlfriend, the death of a loved one, a divorce, or a major family conflict.

Teens who are thinking about suicide might:

- Talk about suicide or death in general
- Give hints that they might not be around anymore
- Talk about feeling hopeless or feeling guilty
- Pull away from friends or family
- Write songs, poems, or letters about death, separation, and loss
- Start giving away treasured possessions to siblings or friends
- Lose the desire to take part in favorite things or activities
- Have trouble concentrating or thinking clearly
- Experience changes in eating or sleeping habits
- Engage in risk-taking behaviors
- Lose interest in school or sports

What Can Parents Do?

Many teens who commit or attempt suicide have given some type of warning to loved ones ahead of time. So it's important for parents to know the warning signs so teens who might be suicidal can get the help they need.

Some adults feel that kids who say they are going to hurt or kill themselves are "just doing it for attention." It's important to realize that if teens are ignored when seeking attention, it may increase the chance of them harming themselves (or worse).

Getting attention in the form of ER visits, doctor's appointments, and residential treatment generally is not something teens want—unless they're seriously depressed and thinking about suicide or at least wishing they were dead. It's important to see warning signs as serious, not as "attention-seeking" to be ignored.

Watch And Listen

Keep a close eye on a teen who is depressed and withdrawn. Understanding depression in teens is very important since it can look different from commonly held beliefs about depression. For example, it may take the form of problems with friends, grades, sleep, or being cranky and irritable rather than chronic sadness or crying.

It's important to try to keep the lines of communication open and express your concern, support, and love. If your teen confides in you, show that you take those concerns seriously. A fight with a friend might not seem like a big deal to you in the larger scheme of things, but for a teen it can feel immense and consuming. It's important not to minimize or discount what your teen is going through, as this can increase his or her sense of hopelessness.

If your teen doesn't feel comfortable talking with you, suggest a more neutral person, such as another relative, a clergy member, a coach, a school counselor, or your child's doctor.

Ask Questions

Some parents are reluctant to ask teens if they have been thinking about suicide or hurting themselves. Some fear that by asking, they will plant the idea of suicide in their teen's head.

It's always a good idea to ask, even though doing so can be difficult. Sometimes it helps to explain why you're asking. For instance, you might say: "I've noticed that you've been talking a lot about wanting to be dead. Have you been having thoughts about trying to kill yourself?"

Get Help

If you learn that your child is thinking about suicide, get help immediately. Your doctor can refer you to a psychologist or psychiatrist, or your local hospital's department of psychiatry can provide a list of doctors in your area. Your local mental health association or county medical society can also provide references. In an emergency, you can call (800) SUICIDE or (800) 999-9999.

If your teen is in a crisis situation, your local emergency room can conduct a comprehensive psychiatric evaluation and refer you to the appropriate resources. If you're unsure about whether you should bring your child to the emergency room, contact your doctor or call (800) SUICIDE for help.

If you've scheduled an appointment with a mental health professional, make sure to keep the appointment, even if your teen says he or she is feeling better or doesn't want to go. Suicidal thoughts do tend to come and go; however, it is important that your teen get help developing the skills necessary to decrease the likelihood that suicidal thoughts and behaviors will emerge again if a crisis arises.

If You've Lost A Child To Suicide

For parents, the death of a child is the most painful loss imaginable. For parents who've lost a child to suicide, the pain and grief can be intensified. Although these feelings may never completely go away, survivors of suicide can take steps to begin the healing process:

- Maintain contact with others. Suicide can be a very isolating experience for surviving family members because friends often don't know what to say or how to help. Seek out supportive people to talk with about your child and your feelings. If those around you seem uncomfortable about reaching out, initiate the conversation and ask for their help.

- Remember that your other family members are grieving, too, and that everyone expresses grief in their own way. Your other children, in particular, may try to deal with their pain alone so as not to burden you with additional worries. Be there for each other through the tears, anger, and silences—and, if necessary, seek help and support together.

- Expect that anniversaries, birthdays, and holidays may be difficult. Important days and holidays often reawaken a sense of loss and anxiety. On those days, do what's best for your emotional needs, whether that means surrounding yourself with family and friends or planning a quiet day of reflection.

- Understand that it's normal to feel guilty and to question how this could have happened, but it's also important to realize that you might never get the answers you seek. The healing that takes place over time comes from reaching a point of forgiveness—for both your child and yourself.

- Counseling and support groups can play a tremendous role in helping you to realize you are not alone. Some bereaved family members become part of the suicide prevention network that helps parents, teenagers, and schools learn how to help prevent future tragedies.

[**Ed. Note:** Although this information addresses parents, teens coping with the loss of a friend or sibling may also find the suggestions helpful.]

If your teen refuses to go to the appointment, discuss this with the mental health professional—and consider attending the session and working with the clinician to make sure your teen has access to the help needed. The clinician also might be able to help you devise strategies to help your teen want to get help.

Remember that ongoing conflicts between a parent and child can fuel the fire for a teen who is feeling isolated, misunderstood, devalued, or suicidal. Get help to air family problems and resolve them in a constructive way. Also let the mental health professional know if there is a history of depression, substance abuse, family violence, or other stresses at home, such as an ongoing environment of criticism.

Helping Teens Cope With Loss

What should you do if someone your teen knows, perhaps a family member, friend, or a classmate, has attempted or committed suicide? First, acknowledge your child's many emotions. Some teens say they feel guilty—especially those who felt they could have interpreted their friend's actions and words better.

Others say they feel angry with the person who committed or attempted suicide for having done something so selfish. Still others say they feel no strong emotions or don't know how to express how they feel. Reassure your child that there is no right or wrong way to feel, and that it's OK to talk about it when he or she feels ready.

When someone attempts suicide and survives, people might be afraid of or uncomfortable talking with him or her about it. Tell your teen to resist this urge; this is a time when a person absolutely needs to feel connected to others.

Many schools address a student's suicide by calling in special counselors to talk with the students and help them cope. If your teen is dealing with a friend or classmate's suicide, encourage him or her to make use of these resources or to talk to you or another trusted adult.

Part Four
Diseases And Disorders With A
Possible Stress Component

Chapter 32

Asthma

Stress And Asthma

Stress is a common asthma trigger. Stress and anxiety sometimes make you feel short of breath and may cause your asthma symptoms to become worse.

You cannot avoid stress; it is part of daily life. However, developing effective ways to manage stress and learning to relax can help you prevent shortness of breath and avoid panic.

Here are some ways to manage stress:

- **Learn to change thought patterns that produce stress.** What you think, how you think, what you expect, and what you tell yourself often determine how you feel and how well you manage rising stress levels.

- **Reduce stressors (causes of stress).** Identify the major stressors in your life: money problems, relationship problems, grief, too many deadlines, busy schedule, and lack of support. If you can't resolve these stressors alone, get professional help for problems that are too difficult to deal with by yourself.

- **Try to avoid situations that trigger stress for you.** Practice effective time-management skills, such as delegating when appropriate, setting priorities, pacing yourself, and taking time out for yourself.

- **Practice relaxation exercises.** Relaxation exercises are simple to perform and combine deep breathing, releasing of muscle tension, and clearing of negative thoughts. If you practice these exercises regularly, you can use them when needed to lessen the negative effects of stress.

  Relaxation exercises include diaphragmatic and pursed lip breathing, imagery, repetitive phrases (repeating a phrase that triggers a physical relaxation, such as "Relax and let go"), and progressive muscle relaxation. Many commercial audiotapes and books that teach these exercises are available.

- **Exercise!** It's an excellent way to burn off the accumulated effects of stress.

- **Get enough sleep.** If you are not sleeping well, you will have less energy and fewer resources for coping with stress. Developing good sleep habits is very important. Here are some tips:

  - Do not go to bed until you are tired.

  - Develop specific bedtime rituals and stick to them.

  - If you have trouble sleeping, do not watch TV, read, or eat in bed.

  - Do not engage in exercise or strenuous activity immediately before bedtime.

  - Avoid caffeine.

  - Do not nap.

  - Go to bed and get up at the same time every day, including on the weekends.

- **Follow the recommended nutritional guidelines.** Junk food and refined sugars low in nutritional value and high in calories can leave you feeling out of energy and sluggish. Limiting sugar, caffeine, and alcohol can promote health and reduce stress.

- **Delegate responsibility.** Stress overload often results from having too many responsibilities. You can free up time and decrease stress by delegating responsibilities. Take a team approach and involve everyone in sharing the load. Try applying these guidelines at home or modifying them to fit your situation at work:

  - Make a list of the types of tasks involved in the job.

  - Take time to train someone to do the job or specific tasks.

  - Assign responsibility to a specific person.

  - Rotate unpleasant duties.

- Give clear, specific instructions with deadlines.

- Be appreciative; let people know you are pleased by a job well done. Allow others to do a job their own way.

- Give up being a perfectionist.

- **Seek support from your family.** The support of family and friends is very important. Social support is the single most important buffer against stress. Here are some tips you can offer to your family or friends when they ask you how they can help. Family and friends can:

  - Help you remain as active and independent as possible.

  - Provide emotional support.

  - Help with household chores and with grocery shopping and other errands as necessary.

  - Learn what they can about your condition and prescribed treatment by attending doctors' appointments with you.

  - Provide encouragement and help you follow your prescribed treatment plan.

Chapter 33

Back Pain And Emotional Distress

Common Reactions To Back Pain

Four out of five adults will experience an episode of significant back pain sometime during their life. Not surprisingly, back pain is one of the problems most often seen by health care providers. Fortunately, the majority of patients with back pain will successfully recover and return to normal social and work activities within 2–4 months, often without treatment.

In 1979, the major professional organization specializing in pain—the International Association for the Study of Pain—introduced the most widely used definition of pain: "an unpleasant sensory and emotional experience associated with actual or potential damage, or described in terms of such damage." This pain is a complex experience that includes both physical and psychological factors.

It is quite normal to have emotional reactions to acute back pain. These reactions can include fear, anxiety, and worry about what the pain means, how long it will last, and how much it will interfere with activities of daily living. Though it's normal to avoid activity that causes pain, complete inactivity is ill-advised. Rather, it is important to take an active role in managing pain by participating in physician-guided activities.

There are now accepted clinical guidelines for management of acute back pain (by definition, within the first 10 weeks of pain) and its associated stress. These guidelines emphasize:

- Addressing patients' fears and misconceptions about back pain;
- Providing a reasonable explanation for the pain as well as an expected outcome; and

- Empowering the patient to resume/restore normal activities of daily living through simple prescribed exercises and graded activity.

- This should be supplemented, when necessary, by complementary treatments such as analgesic medications, manual therapy and/or physical therapy for symptomatic relief.

Questions You Need To Ask

In order to minimize emotional distress, it is important to ask your health care provider questions about your back pain so you do not leave the office uncertain or anxious. Understanding your pain will help decrease your anxiety. Keep in mind that, if your pain lasts more than 2–4 months (which is usually considered a normal healing time for most back problems), your condition may become chronic. Chronic pain can be associated with even greater psychological distress.

During the acute period, feelings of helplessness, stress, and even anger towards your health care provider (for not relieving your pain) may occur. In order to help allay this distress, you need to be sure that your health care provider is attending to all of your important physical and psychological needs. You and your health care provider should do the following:

- You should express your concerns about your pain symptoms. It is normal for patients to fear serious disease or disability. Be certain that your health care provider addresses your fears through appropriate medical evaluation and explanation.

- Be certain that your health care provider fully explains what is being looked for or ruled out during these evaluations and tests, and make sure you get the results in terms you can understand.

- If your health care provider recommends staying active, be certain that he or she discusses with you how to stay active safely.

- Inform your health care provider of any functional difficulties your pain is causing (e.g., problems with bending, lifting, etc.) and identify with him or her ways to overcome these difficulties. Also have your health care provider address any problems you have performing your normal work activities.

- The information you receive about your diagnosis and prognosis should be clear to you. Make sure you understand the natural progression of back pain, what "improvement" can be expected, and when it is likely to occur.

- Whenever any recommendations are made, be sure that you or your health care provider writes them down so you can review them after leaving the office.

All of these recommendations are intended to reduce the emotional concerns and stress most patients experience with pain. If you are not satisfied with the treatment and explanations you receive, consider getting a second opinion from another health care provider. Anxiety and stress can actually increase your pain and reduce your pain coping skills.

Relationship Between Stress And Pain

It is important to remember that there is a dynamic relationship between your state of mind (e.g., stress level) and your physical condition (e.g., pain). Pain can cause stress, which causes more pain, which causes more stress, and so on. The more chronic this vicious cycle becomes, the more likely your emotional distress will increase. This cycle can be very difficult to break.

Emotional suffering can lead to loss of sleep, inability to work, as well as feeling irritable and helpless about what can be done. You may feel desperate and attempt to relieve the pain at any cost including the use of invasive medical procedures. Although invasive approaches may be beneficial for some conditions (such as a herniated disc), often they can be avoided if stress and pain are managed at an early point in time.

Education and reassurance from your health care provider goes a long way in preventing or relieving a great deal of stress and anxiety. You also need to be proactive about your condition and treatment. These naturally occurring feelings of anxiety and stress may cloud your judgment. Your goal is to avoid getting into a chronic pain cycle. Reassurance from your health care provider that the pain is only temporary can go a long way to help you avoid becoming preoccupied with pain, and prevent unnecessary worry about the symptoms.

Psychological Interventions For Back Pain

Fortunately, there are a number of psychological therapies that have been successfully used in the management of pain and anxiety. These include stress management, relaxation training, biofeedback, hypnosis, and cognitive-behavioral therapy (a method to reduce feelings of doom and helplessness). There are also medications available to help with sleep problems, anxiety, and depression. Such comprehensive pain management programs, when integrated with your medical care, have proven to be quite successful.

Your health care provider can refer you to a psychological management program if it is appropriate. Participation in such a program does not mean the pain is "all in your head"—it is meant to teach you methods to cope with and control the pain. Remember, pain is a complex experience that includes a close interaction of physical and psychological factors! But together, you and your health care provider can help you manage and overcome your pain.

Chapter 34

Chronic Fatigue Syndrome

What is chronic fatigue syndrome (CFS)?

A person with chronic fatigue syndrome (CFS) feels completely worn out and over-tired. This extreme tiredness makes it hard to do the daily tasks that most of us do without thinking—like dressing, bathing, or eating. Sleep or rest does not make the tiredness go away. It can be made worse by moving, exercising, or even thinking.

CFS can happen over time or come on suddenly. People who get CFS over time get more and more tired over weeks or months. People who get CFS suddenly feel fine one day and then feel extremely tired the next. A person with CFS may have muscle pain, trouble focusing, or insomnia (not being able to sleep). The extreme tiredness may come and go. In some cases the extreme tiredness never goes away. The extreme tiredness must go on for at least six months before a diagnosis of CFS can be made.

What causes CFS?

No one knows for sure what causes CFS. Many people with CFS say it started after an infection, such as a cold or stomach bug. It also can follow infection with the Epstein-Barr virus. This is the same virus that causes infectious mononucleosis (sometimes called "mono"). Some people with CFS say it started after a time of great stress, such as the loss of a loved one or major surgery.

About This Chapter: Information in this chapter is excerpted from "Chronic Fatigue Syndrome: Frequently Asked Questions," U.S. Department of Health and Human Services, Office on Women's Health (www.womenshealth.gov), September 2009.

It can be hard to figure out if a person has CFS because extreme tiredness is a common symptom of many illnesses. Also, some medical treatments, such as chemotherapy, can cause extreme tiredness.

What are the signs of CFS?

The signs of CFS can come and go or they can stay with a person. At first, you may feel like you have the flu. As well as extreme tiredness and weakness, main CFS symptoms include:

- Feeling very tired for more than a day (24 hours) after physical or mental exercise

- Forgetting things or having a hard time focusing

- Feeling tired even after sleeping

- Muscle pain or aches

- Pain or aches in joints without swelling or redness

- Headaches of a new type, pattern, or strength

- Tender lymph nodes in the neck or under the arm

- Sore throat

The symptoms above are the main signs of CFS. CFS symptoms may also include:

- Visual disturbances (blurring, sensitivity to light, eye pain)

- Psychological symptoms (irritability, mood swings, panic attacks, anxiety)

- Chills and night sweats

- Low grade fever or low body temperature

- Irritable bowel

- Allergies and sensitivities to foods, odors, chemicals, medications, and noise/sound

- Numbness, tingling, or burning sensations in the face, hands, or feet

- Difficulty sitting or standing straight up, dizziness, balance problems, and fainting

Symptoms of CFS vary widely from person to person and may be serious or mild. Most symptoms cannot be seen by others, which makes it hard for friends, family members, and the public to understand the challenges a person with CFS faces. If you think you may have CFS, talk to your doctor.

Chronic Fatigue Syndrome: General Information

Chronic fatigue syndrome, or CFS, is a devastating and complex disorder. People with CFS have overwhelming fatigue and a host of other symptoms that are not improved by bed rest and that can get worse after physical activity or mental exertion. They often function at a substantially lower level of activity than they were capable of before they became ill.

Besides severe fatigue, other symptoms include muscle pain, impaired memory or mental concentration, insomnia, and post-exertion malaise lasting more than 24 hours. In some cases, CFS can persist for years.

Researchers have not yet identified what causes CFS, and there are no tests to diagnose CFS. Moreover, because many illnesses have fatigue as a symptom, doctors need to take care to rule out other conditions, which may be treatable.

Source: Excerpted from "General Information: Chronic Fatigue Syndrome," Centers for Disease Control and Prevention (www.cdc.gov), May 2012.

How common is CFS? Who gets it?

Experts think at least one million Americans have CFS. Fewer than 20 percent of these cases have been diagnosed, however.

Women are four times as likely as men to develop CFS. The illness occurs most often in people ages 40–59. Still, people of all ages can get CFS. CFS is less common in children than in adults. Studies suggest that CFS occurs more often in adolescents than in children under the age of 12.

CFS occurs in all ethnic groups and races, and in countries around the world. People of all income levels can develop CFS, although there is evidence that it is more common in lower-income than in higher-income persons. CFS is sometimes seen in members of the same family, but there is no evidence that it is contagious. Instead, it may run in families because of a genetic link. Further research is needed to explore how this happens.

How would my doctor know if I have CFS?

It can be hard for your doctor to diagnose CFS because there is no lab test for it. Also, many signs of CFS are also signs of other illnesses—or side effects of medical treatments. All cases are diagnosed by the 1994 Centers for Disease Control (CDC) definition, which is also sometimes called the "Fukuda criteria" after the name of a leading researcher in the field. Children with CFS can be diagnosed by a new pediatric case definition, which differs from the adult definition.

If you think you may have CFS, see your doctor. Your doctor will:

- Ask you about your physical and mental health;

- Do a physical exam;

- Order urine and blood tests, which will tell your doctor if something other than CFS might be causing your symptoms;

- Order more tests, if your urine and blood tests do not show a cause for your symptoms; and

- Classify you as having CFS if:

    - You have been extremely tired for six months or more and tests do not show a cause for your symptoms; and

    - You have four or more of the symptoms listed in the section, "What are the signs of CFS?" in this chapter.

Childhood Adversity As A Risk Factor For Adult Chronic Fatigue Syndrome

It is a well-established fact that experiences during early life shape the development of the brain, particularly during sensitive periods. Adverse experiences can "program" the development of certain brain regions that are involved in the regulation and integration of hormonal, autonomic, and immune responses to challenges later in life. Such challenges may encompass infections, physical stresses, or emotional challenges.

Approximately 14 percent of children in the U.S. are subjected to some form of maltreatment, and in 2007, over three million reports of childhood abuse and neglect were investigated. Childhood trauma, defined as abuse, neglect, or loss, is a stressor that affects the physical and mental well-being of humans from infancy throughout the lifespan. In various animal and human studies, childhood trauma has been associated with low resting cortisol levels, altered stress response, increased inflammatory markers, and cognitive impairment.

Childhood abuse has been connected to a wide range of disorders, such as depression, anxiety disorders, and substance abuse problems, but also more classic medical diseases such as cardiovascular disease. Of note, markedly elevated levels of pain and fatigue have been reported in studies of survivors of childhood abuse.

Chronic fatigue syndrome (CFS) is a debilitating illness that can sometimes occur in response to a stressor or a challenge. For example, there have been reports of people developing CFS after being in a serious car accident. Other examples of challenges are increased rates of CFS in Gulf war veterans and triggered relapses of CFS in persons affected by Hurricane Andrew.

This process can take a long time (even years), so try to be patient with your doctor. While these tests are being done, talk to your doctor about ways to help ease your symptoms. Although CFS is not a form of depression, many patients develop depression as a result of dealing with a long-term illness.

How is CFS treated?

Right now, there is no cure for CFS. But there are things you can do to feel better. Talk to your doctor about ways to ease your symptoms and deal with your tiredness, which may include lifestyle changes and medications.

Lifestyle Changes

- Try to stop or do less of the things that seem to trigger your tiredness. For a week or two write down what you do each day. Note when you feel really tired. Then, look over this list to find out which activities tend to tire you out. An occupational therapist can help

Upon stress exposure, our central nervous system will activate hormone and immune responses that help the body to maintain balance during stress. There is evidence that childhood maltreatment may alter the way the body's regulatory systems respond to stress. Early adversity may thus increase a person's risk to develop adult CFS, particularly in response to challenges. Therefore, childhood trauma may be an important risk factor for adult CFS. Research has shown that when adults (with CFS and without CFS) were asked about childhood trauma, those with CFS self-reported higher levels of childhood maltreatment. In particular, for women, emotional and sexual abuse during childhood was associated with a greater risk of developing CFS later in life.

Of note, a risk factor is not "the cause" of a disorder; it increases the relative risk, but is not present in all cases. The cause of CFS is still unknown, but childhood trauma might be a factor that contributes to adult CFS risk in a subset of people. While these findings are important, and have the potential to help many people, it is important to realize that not all persons with adult CFS experienced maltreatment as a child. Childhood maltreatment is just one risk factor for CFS and does not explain how other people with CFS (who did not experience such trauma) developed the illness.

The results from this research are important because healthcare providers can help people with a history of childhood maltreatment. For some people that have both a past of childhood maltreatment and CFS, talk therapy may be beneficial. While more research is needed on CFS and childhood maltreatment, patients are encouraged to talk to their healthcare provider about their physical and mental health history.

Source: "Childhood Adversity as a Risk Factor for Adult CFS," Centers for Disease Control and Prevention (www.cdc.gov), October 2011.

you by looking at your daily habits and suggesting changes to help you save energy. Your doctor can help you find an occupational therapist near where you live.

- At the end of the day, try thinking about how much energy you think you had that day, and how much energy you actually used that day. If you keep these two amounts of energy similar over time, you may slowly gain more strength and energy. Think about which activities are most important to you, and which activities you do not need to do as often. Make sure to tell other people in your life how much energy you can actually use each day. They can help make sure you don't do too much. It is important to remember that energy can mean mental, emotional, or physical energy.

Medications

- Over-the-counter pain relievers such as Advil, Motrin, or Aleve can help with body aches, headaches, and muscle and joint pain.

- Non-drowsy antihistamines (an-tee-HISS-tah-meens) can help with allergy symptoms, such as runny nose and itchy eyes.

- Prescription medications like doxepin (DOCKS-ih-pin) or amitriptyline (am-ih-TRIP-tah-leen) can help improve sleep.

Some people say their CFS symptoms get better with complementary or alternative treatments, such as massage, acupuncture, chiropractic care, yoga, stretching, or self-hypnosis. Keep in mind that many alternative treatments, dietary supplements, and herbal remedies claim to cure CFS, but they might do more harm than good. Talk to your doctor before seeing someone else for treatment or before trying alternative therapies.

Also, keep in mind that your doctor may need to learn more about CFS to better help you. If you feel your doctor doesn't know a lot about CFS, or has doubts about it being a "real" illness, see another doctor for a second opinion. Contact a local university medical school or research center for help finding a doctor who treats people with CFS.

Chapter 35

Fibromyalgia

Fibromyalgia syndrome is a common and chronic disorder characterized by widespread pain, diffuse tenderness, and a number of other symptoms. The word "fibromyalgia" comes from the Latin term for fibrous tissue (fibro) and the Greek ones for muscle (myo) and pain (algia).

Although fibromyalgia is often considered an arthritis-related condition, it is not truly a form of arthritis (a disease of the joints) because it does not cause inflammation or damage to the joints, muscles, or other tissues. Like arthritis, however, fibromyalgia can cause significant pain and fatigue, and it can interfere with a person's ability to carry on daily activities. Also like arthritis, fibromyalgia is considered a rheumatic condition, a medical condition that impairs the joints and/or soft tissues and causes chronic pain.

In addition to pain and fatigue, people who have fibromyalgia may experience a variety of other symptoms including:

- Cognitive and memory problems (sometimes referred to as "fibro fog")
- Sleep disturbances
- Morning stiffness
- Headaches
- Irritable bowel syndrome
- Painful menstrual periods
- Numbness or tingling of the extremities

About This Chapter: Information in this chapter is excerpted from "Questions and Answers About Fibromyalgia," National Institute of Arthritis and Musculoskeletal and Skin Diseases (www.niams.nih.gov), July 2011.

- Restless legs syndrome

- Temperature sensitivity

- Sensitivity to loud noises or bright lights

Fibromyalgia is a syndrome rather than a disease. A syndrome is a collection of signs, symptoms, and medical problems that tend to occur together but are not related to a specific, identifiable cause. A disease, on the other hand, has a specific cause or causes and recognizable signs and symptoms.

Who gets fibromyalgia?

Scientists estimate that fibromyalgia affects five million Americans age 18 or older. For unknown reasons, between 80 and 90 percent of those diagnosed with fibromyalgia are women; however, men and children also can be affected. Most people are diagnosed during middle age, although the symptoms often become present earlier in life.

Several studies indicate that women who have a family member with fibromyalgia are more likely to have fibromyalgia themselves, but the exact reason for this—whether it be heredity, shared environmental factors, or both—is unknown. One current study supported by the National Institute of Arthritis and Musculoskeletal and Skin Diseases (NIAMS) is trying to determine whether variations in certain genes cause some people to be more sensitive to stimuli, which leads to pain syndromes.

What causes fibromyalgia?

The causes of fibromyalgia are unknown, but there are probably a number of factors involved. Many people associate the development of fibromyalgia with a physically or emotionally stressful or traumatic event, such as an automobile accident. Some connect it to repetitive injuries. Others link it to an illness. For others, fibromyalgia seems to occur spontaneously.

Many researchers are examining other causes, including problems with how the central nervous system (the brain and spinal cord) processes pain. Some scientists speculate that a person's genes may regulate the way his or her body processes painful stimuli. According to this theory, people with fibromyalgia may have a gene or genes that cause them to react strongly to stimuli that most people would not perceive as painful.

How is fibromyalgia diagnosed?

Research shows that people with fibromyalgia typically see many doctors before receiving the diagnosis. One reason for this may be that pain and fatigue, the main symptoms of fibromyalgia, overlap with those of many other conditions. Therefore, doctors often have to rule out other potential causes of these symptoms before making a diagnosis of fibromyalgia. Another reason is that there are currently no diagnostic laboratory tests for fibromyalgia; standard laboratory tests fail to reveal a physiologic reason for pain. Because there is no generally accepted, objective test for fibromyalgia, some doctors unfortunately may conclude a patient's pain is not real, or they may tell the patient there is little they can do. A doctor familiar with fibromyalgia, however, can make a diagnosis based on criteria established by the American College of Rheumatology (ACR).

How is fibromyalgia treated?

Fibromyalgia can be difficult to treat. Not all doctors are familiar with fibromyalgia and its treatment, so it is important to find a doctor who is. Many family physicians, general internists, or rheumatologists (doctors who specialize in arthritis and other conditions that affect the joints or soft tissues) can treat fibromyalgia.

Fibromyalgia treatment often requires a team approach, with your doctor, a physical therapist, possibly other health professionals, and most importantly, yourself, all playing an active role. It can be hard to assemble this team, and you may struggle to find the right professionals to treat you. When you do, however, the combined expertise of these various professionals can help you improve your quality of life.

Only three medications, duloxetine (Cymbalta), milnacipran (Savella), and pregabalin (Lyrica) are approved by the U.S. Food and Drug Administration (FDA) for the treatment of fibromyalgia. Cymbalta was originally developed for and is still used to treat depression. Savella is similar to a drug used to treat depression, but is FDA approved only for fibromyalgia. Lyrica is a medication developed to treat neuropathic pain (chronic pain caused by damage to the nervous system).

Following are some of the most commonly used categories of drugs for fibromyalgia.

Analgesics: Analgesics are painkillers. They range from over-the-counter acetaminophen (Tylenol) to prescription medicines, such as tramadol (Ultram), and even stronger narcotic preparations. For a subset of people with fibromyalgia, narcotic medications are prescribed for severe muscle pain, however there is no solid evidence showing that for most people narcotics actually work to treat the chronic pain of fibromyalgia.

Nonsteroidal Anti-Inflammatory Drugs (NSAIDs): As their name implies, nonsteroidal anti-inflammatory drugs, including aspirin, ibuprofen (Advil, Motrin), and naproxen sodium (Anaprox, Aleve), are used to treat inflammation. Although inflammation is not a symptom of fibromyalgia, NSAIDs also relieve pain. The drugs work by inhibiting substances in the body called prostaglandins, which play a role in pain and inflammation. These medications, some of which are available without a prescription, may help ease the muscle aches of fibromyalgia.

Antidepressants: Perhaps the most useful medications for fibromyalgia are several in the antidepressant class. These drugs work equally well in fibromyalgia patients with and without depression, because antidepressants elevate the levels of certain chemicals in the brain (including serotonin and norepinephrine) that are associated not only with depression, but also with pain and fatigue. Increasing the levels of these chemicals can reduce pain in people who have fibromyalgia.

Benzodiazepines: Benzodiazepines can sometimes help people with fibromyalgia by relaxing tense, painful muscles and stabilizing the erratic brain waves that can interfere with deep sleep. Benzodiazepines also can relieve the symptoms of restless legs syndrome, a neurological disorder that is more common among people with fibromyalgia. The disorder is characterized by unpleasant sensations in the legs and an uncontrollable urge to move the legs, particularly when at rest, in an effort to relieve these feelings. Doctors usually prescribe benzodiazepines only for people who have not responded to other therapies because of the potential for addiction.

Other Medications: In addition to the previously described general categories of drugs, doctors may recommend or prescribe others, depending on a person's specific symptoms or fibromyalgia-related conditions (for example, for people with irritable bowel syndrome, doctors may suggest fiber supplements or laxatives to relieve constipation). Antispasmodic medications may be useful for relieving intestinal spasms and reducing abdominal pain. Other symptom-specific medications include sleep medications, muscle relaxants, and headache remedies.

People with fibromyalgia also may benefit from a combination of physical and occupational therapy, from learning pain management and coping techniques, and from properly balancing rest and activity.

Complementary And Alternative Therapies: Many people with fibromyalgia also report varying degrees of success with complementary and alternative therapies, including massage, movement therapies (such as Pilates and the Feldenkrais method), chiropractic treatments, acupuncture, and various herbs and dietary supplements for different fibromyalgia symptoms.

Although some of these supplements are being studied for fibromyalgia, there is little, if any, scientific proof yet that they help. If you would like to try a complementary or alternative therapy, you should first speak with your doctor.

Will fibromyalgia get better with time?

Fibromyalgia is a chronic condition, meaning it lasts a long time—possibly a lifetime. However, it may be comforting to know that fibromyalgia is not a progressive disease. It is never fatal, and it will not cause damage to the joints, muscles, or internal organs. In many people, the condition does improve over time.

What can I do to try to feel better?

Besides taking medicine prescribed by your doctor, there are many things you can do to minimize the impact of fibromyalgia on your life. These include:

- **Get enough sleep.** Getting enough sleep and the right kind of sleep can help ease the pain and fatigue of fibromyalgia.

- **Exercise.** Although pain and fatigue may make exercise and daily activities difficult, it is crucial to be as physically active as possible. Research has repeatedly shown that regular exercise is one of the most effective treatments for fibromyalgia.

Tips For Good Sleep

- **Keep regular sleep habits.** Try to get to bed at the same time and get up at the same time every day—even on weekends and vacations.

- **Avoid caffeine in the late afternoon and evening.** If consumed too close to bedtime, the caffeine in coffee, soft drinks, chocolate, and some medications can keep you from sleeping or sleeping soundly.

- **Time your exercise.** Regular daytime exercise can improve nighttime sleep. But avoid exercising within three hours of bedtime, which actually can be stimulating, keeping you awake.

- **Avoid daytime naps.** Sleeping in the afternoon can interfere with nighttime sleep. If you feel you cannot get by without a nap, set an alarm for one hour.

- **Reserve your bed for sleeping.** Watching the late news, reading a suspense novel, or working on your laptop in bed can stimulate you, making it hard to sleep.

- **Keep your bedroom dark, quiet, and cool.**

- **Avoid liquids and spicy meals before bed.** Heartburn and late night trips to the bathroom are not conducive to good sleep.

- **Wind down before bed.** Avoid working right up to bedtime. Do relaxing activities, such as listening to soft music or taking a warm bath, that get you ready to sleep.

- **Make changes at work.** Most people with fibromyalgia continue to work, but they may have to make big changes to do so. For example, some people cut down the number of hours they work, switch to a less demanding job, or adapt a current job.

- **Eat well.** Although some people with fibromyalgia report feeling better when they eat or avoid certain foods, no specific diet has been proven to influence fibromyalgia. Of course, it is important to have a healthy, balanced diet. Not only will proper nutrition give you more energy and make you generally feel better, it will also help you avoid other health problems.

What are researchers learning about fibromyalgia?

The research on fibromyalgia supported by NIAMS covers a broad spectrum, ranging from basic laboratory research to studies of medications and interventions designed to encourage behaviors that reduce pain and change behaviors that worsen or perpetuate pain.

Chapter 36

Multiple Sclerosis

Multiple sclerosis (MS) is the most common disabling neurological disease of young adults. It most often appears when people are between 20–40 years old. However, it can also affect children and older people.

The course of MS is unpredictable. A small number of those with MS will have a mild course with little to no disability, while another smaller group will have a steadily worsening disease that leads to increased disability over time. Most people with MS, however, will have short periods of symptoms followed by long stretches of relative relief, with partial or full recovery. There is no way to predict, at the beginning, how an individual person's disease will progress.

Researchers have spent decades trying to understand why some people get MS and others don't, and why some individuals with MS have symptoms that progress rapidly while others do not. How does the disease begin? Why is the course of MS so different from person to person? Is there anything we can do to prevent it? Can it be cured?

This chapter includes information about why MS develops, how it progresses, and what new therapies are being used to treat its symptoms and slow its progression. New treatments can reduce long-term disability for many people with MS. However, there are still no cures and no clear ways to prevent MS from developing.

What is multiple sclerosis?

MS is a neuroinflammatory disease that affects myelin, a substance that makes up the membrane that wraps around nerve fibers—commonly called white matter. Researchers have

About This Chapter: This chapter begins with excerpts from "Multiple Sclerosis: Hope Through Research," National Institute of Neurological Disorders and Stroke (www.ninds.nih.gov), August 2012. Additional information from the National Multiple Sclerosis Society concerning MS and stress is cited separately within the chapter.

learned that MS also damages the nerve cell bodies, which are found in the brain's gray matter, as well as the axons themselves in the brain, spinal cord, and optic nerve (the nerve that transmits visual information from the eye to the brain). As the disease progresses, the brain's cortex shrinks.

The term multiple sclerosis refers to the distinctive areas of scar tissue (sclerosis or plaques) that are visible in the white matter of people who have MS. Plaques can be as small as a pinhead or as large as the size of a golf ball. Doctors can see these areas by examining the brain and spinal cord using a type of brain scan called magnetic resonance imaging (MRI).

While MS sometimes causes severe disability, it is only rarely fatal and most people with MS have a normal life expectancy.

What are plaques made of and why do they develop?

Plaques, or lesions, are the result of an inflammatory process in the brain that causes immune system cells to attack myelin. The myelin sheath helps to speed nerve impulses traveling within the nervous system. Axons are also damaged in MS, although not as extensively, or as early in the disease, as myelin.

Under normal circumstances, cells of the immune system travel in and out of the brain patrolling for infectious agents (viruses, for example) or unhealthy cells. This is called the "surveillance" function of the immune system.

Surveillance cells usually won't spring into action unless they recognize an infectious agent or unhealthy cells. When they do, they produce substances to stop the infectious agent. If they encounter unhealthy cells, they either kill them directly or clean out the dying area and produce substances that promote healing and repair among the cells that are left.

Researchers have observed that immune cells behave differently in the brains of people with MS. They become active and attack what appears to be healthy myelin. It is unclear what triggers this attack. MS is one of many autoimmune disorders, such as rheumatoid arthritis and lupus, in which the immune system mistakenly attacks a person's healthy tissue as opposed to performing its normal role of attacking foreign invaders like viruses and bacteria. Whatever the reason, during these periods of immune system activity, most of the myelin within the affected area is damaged or destroyed. The axons also may be damaged. The symptoms of MS depend on the severity of the immune reaction as well as the location and extent of the plaques, which primarily appear in the brain stem, cerebellum, spinal cord, optic nerves, and the white matter of the brain around the brain ventricles (fluid-filled spaces inside of the brain).

What are the signs and symptoms of MS?

The symptoms of MS usually begin over one to several days, but in some forms, they may develop more slowly. They may be mild or severe and may go away quickly or last for months. Sometimes the initial symptoms of MS are overlooked because they disappear in a day or so and normal function returns. Because symptoms come and go in the majority of people with MS, the presence of symptoms is called an attack, or in medical terms, an exacerbation. Recovery from symptoms is referred to as remission, while a return of symptoms is called a relapse. This form of MS is therefore called relapsing-remitting MS, in contrast to a more slowly developing form called primary progressive MS. Progressive MS can also be a second stage of the illness that follows years of relapsing-remitting symptoms.

A diagnosis of MS is often delayed because MS shares symptoms with other neurological conditions and diseases.

The first symptoms of MS often include:

- Vision problems such as blurred or double vision or optic neuritis, which causes pain in the eye and a rapid loss of vision
- Weak, stiff muscles, often with painful muscle spasms
- Tingling or numbness in the arms, legs, trunk of the body, or face
- Clumsiness, particularly difficulty staying balanced when walking
- Bladder control problems, either inability to control the bladder or urgency
- Dizziness that doesn't go away

MS may also cause later symptoms such as:

- Mental or physical fatigue, which accompanies the above symptoms during an attack
- Mood changes, such as depression or euphoria
- Changes in the ability to concentrate or to multitask effectively
- Difficulty making decisions, planning, or prioritizing at work or in private life

People with MS, especially those who have had the disease for a long time, can experience difficulty with thinking, learning, memory, and judgment. The first signs of what doctors call cognitive dysfunction may be subtle. The person may have problems finding the right word to say, or trouble remembering how to do routine tasks on the job or at home. Day-to-day decisions, that once came easily, may now be made more slowly and show poor judgment. Changes may be so small or happen so slowly that it takes a family member or friend to point them out.

How many people have MS?

No one knows exactly how many people have MS. Experts think there are currently 250,000 to 350,000 people in the United States diagnosed with MS. This estimate suggests that approximately 200 new cases are diagnosed every week. Studies of the prevalence (the proportion of individuals in a population having a particular disease) of MS indicate that the rate of the disease has increased steadily during the twentieth century.

As with most autoimmune disorders, twice as many women are affected by MS as men. MS is more common in colder climates. People of Northern European descent appear to be at the highest risk for the disease, regardless of where they live. Native Americans of North and South America, as well as Asian American populations, have relatively low rates of MS.

What causes MS?

The ultimate cause of MS is damage to myelin, nerve fibers, and neurons in the brain and spinal cord, which together make up the central nervous system (CNS). But how that happens, and why, are questions that challenge researchers. Evidence appears to show that MS is a disease caused by genetic vulnerabilities combined with environmental factors.

Although there is little doubt that the immune system contributes to the brain and spinal cord tissue destruction of MS, the exact target of the immune system attacks and which immune system cells cause the destruction isn't fully understood.

Researchers have several possible explanations for what might be going on. The immune system could be: fighting some kind of infectious agent (for example, a virus) that has components which mimic components of the brain; destroying brain cells because they are unhealthy; and/or mistakenly identifying normal brain cells as foreign.

The last possibility has been the favored explanation for many years. Research now suggests that the first two activities might also play a role in the development of MS. There is a special barrier, called the blood-brain barrier, which separates the brain and spinal cord from the immune system. If there is a break in the barrier, it exposes the brain to the immune system for the first time. When this happens, the immune system may misinterpret the brain as "foreign."

Genetic Susceptibility: Susceptibility to MS may be inherited. Studies of families indicate that relatives of an individual with MS have an increased risk for developing the disease. Experts estimate that about 15 percent of individuals with MS have one or more family members or relatives who also have MS. But even identical twins, whose DNA is exactly the same, have only a one in three chance of both having the disease. This suggests that MS is not entirely controlled by genes.

Sunlight And Vitamin D: A number of studies have suggested that people who spend more time in the sun and those with relatively high levels of vitamin D are less likely to develop MS. Bright sunlight helps human skin produce vitamin D. Researchers believe that vitamin D may help regulate the immune system in ways that reduce the risk of MS. People from regions near the equator, where there is a great deal of bright sunlight, generally have a much lower risk of MS than people from temperate areas such as the United States and Canada. Other studies suggest that people with higher levels of vitamin D generally have less severe MS and fewer relapses.

Smoking: A number of studies have found that people who smoke are more likely to develop MS. People who smoke also tend to have more brain lesions and brain shrinkage than non-smokers.

Infectious Factors And Viruses: A number of viruses have been found in people with MS, but the virus most consistently linked to the development of MS is Epstein Barr virus (EBV), the virus that causes mononucleosis.

Autoimmune And Inflammatory Processes: Tissue inflammation and antibodies in the blood that fight normal components of the body and tissue in people with MS are similar to those found in other autoimmune diseases. Along with overlapping evidence from genetic studies, these findings suggest that MS results from some kind of disturbed regulation of the immune system.

How is MS diagnosed?

There is no single test used to diagnose MS. Doctors use a number of tests to rule out or confirm the diagnosis. There are many other disorders that can mimic MS. Some of these other disorders can be cured, while others require different treatments than those used for MS. Therefore it is very important to perform a thorough investigation before making a diagnosis.

In addition to a complete medical history, physical examination, and a detailed neurological examination, a doctor will order a magnetic resonance imaging (MRI) scan of the head and spine to look for the characteristic lesions of MS.

What is the course of MS?

The course of MS is different for each individual, which makes it difficult to predict. For most people, it starts with a first attack, usually (but not always) followed by a full to almost-full recovery. Weeks, months, or even years may pass before another attack occurs, followed again by a period of relief from symptoms.

What is an exacerbation or attack of MS?

An exacerbation—which is also called a relapse, flare-up, or attack—is a sudden worsening of MS symptoms, or the appearance of new symptoms that lasts for at least 24 hours. MS relapses are thought to be associated with the development of new areas of damage in the brain. Exacerbations are characteristic of relapsing-remitting MS, in which attacks are followed by periods of complete or partial recovery with no apparent worsening of symptoms.

An attack may be mild or its symptoms may be severe enough to significantly interfere with life's daily activities. Most exacerbations last from several days to several weeks, although some have been known to last for months.

When the symptoms of the attack subside, an individual with MS is said to be in remission. However, MRI data have shown that this is somewhat misleading because MS lesions continue to appear during these remission periods.

Are there treatments available for MS?

There is still no cure for MS, but there are treatments for initial attacks, medications and therapies to improve symptoms, and recently developed drugs to slow the worsening of the disease. These new drugs have been shown to reduce the number and severity of relapses and to delay the long term progression of MS.

During the past 20 years, researchers have made major breakthroughs in MS treatment due to new knowledge about the immune system and the ability to use MRI to monitor MS in patients. As a result, a number of medical therapies have been found to reduce relapses in persons with relapsing-remitting MS. These drugs are called disease modulating drugs.

The current FDA-approved therapies for MS are designed to modulate or suppress the inflammatory reactions of the disease. They are most effective for relapsing-remitting MS at early stages of the disease.

How do doctors treat the symptoms of MS?

MS causes a variety of symptoms that can interfere with daily activities but which can usually be treated or managed to reduce their impact. Many of these issues are best treated by neurologists who have advanced training in the treatment of MS and who can prescribe specific medications to treat the problems.

What research is being done?

Although researchers haven't been able to identify the cause of MS with any certainty, there has been excellent progress in other areas of MS research—especially in development of new treatments to prevent exacerbations of the disease. New discoveries are constantly changing treatment options for patients.

MS And Stress

Source: Reprinted from "MS and Stress" by Marcella Durand, *InsideMS*, October/November 2005. Copyright National Multiple Sclerosis Society (www.nationalmssociety.org), 2005. Reprinted with permission. Reviewed by David A. Cooke, MD, FACP, April 2013.

A close friend of mine is planning her wedding. At dinner a few nights ago, while describing the preparations, she became increasingly distraught. Finally she stopped, looked up at me sadly, and sighed, "I guess I just don't handle stress very well."

My first thought was, who does? Whether getting married, starting a new job or leaving an old one, or dealing with the loss of a loved one, life can sometimes seem overwhelming. And being told we need to reduce our stress often makes us feel even more pressured: Taking yoga classes or practicing deep breathing are just more things to add to our to-do list.

Ironically, even though everyone experiences it, stress is difficult to define objectively. "Different people really mean different things when they talk about stress," said Nicholas LaRocca, PhD, the director of Health Care Delivery and Policy Research for the National Multiple Sclerosis Society. "Not just the general public, but scientists, too."

There are many kinds of potentially stressful situations, and each person has his or her own response. One person may be devastated by the loss of a job, while another may find working fulltime stressful. There's everyday stress, like being stuck in traffic, or there's traumatic stress, such as divorce or loss of a child. There are even general stresses brought on by war or terrorism.

Multiple sclerosis brings its own kinds of stress. New York City paramedic Maggie Staiger was diagnosed in August 2001, and a month later she worked as a paramedic at the World Trade Center site. "All these things are happening—you have to give yourself shots, your whole life changes—and then everyone tells you to try not to get stressed out. How in the world are you not supposed to get stressed out?" she said.

Stressing Over Stress

Dr. LaRocca calls it "stress related to worrying about stress." If you think that stress could cause an exacerbation—which has never been definitively proven—then you may stress over managing your stress.

Rosalind Kalb, PhD, director of the Society's Professional Resource Center, agreed. "People can be so worried about anything making their disease worse that it becomes another stress in and of itself." In addition, friends or family members may feel responsible or guilty for causing stress, thinking that they may be worsening a person's MS.

"Issues that need to be discussed sometimes don't come up because a family member is afraid to bring them up," Dr. Kalb said. "Rather than being brought out into the open and re-solved, they get swept under the carpet because the person doesn't want to bring up something that might upset the loved one with MS."

"One idea I find incredibly offensive is the idea that I wouldn't have MS if I'd managed my stress better," Staiger said. "There's the implication that if you can affect it with your mind then it was caused by your mind." She adds, "When I first got diagnosed, and then there was the World Trade Center, I was reading all this stuff about MS that emphasized 'try to avoid stress, try to avoid stress.' I thought, this is horrible! But I realized that, while I can't really avoid stress, I can change my reaction to stress."

The Missing Link

The first thing to know is that while stress can make us feel worse, whether upsetting our stomachs or knotting our neck muscles, no research group has been able to prove between MS and stress. Many have tried.

"There's no doubt that there is a link in a general sense between stress another things that happen to the human body," Dr. LaRocca said. "But what they are and how they operate in each case is not so clear." He added, "People get caught up in this question: Is stress makings worse? I think we need to focus deeper than that and try to define stress in a scientifically rigorous way and then relate it to what's happening to the immune system."

Dr. Kalb agreed. "If people say they feel worse, I believe them, but we just don't know what the mechanism is." It's difficult to separate out the general effects of stress—such as making people feel more tired or jittery—from what actually happens to the immune system when it is under stress. The immune system is made up of many different elements working together, almost like a web. It is a mistake to point to a single factor, like stress, and blame it for everything.

"It's important for people with MS to know that there have been a lot of studies, but we still don't have conclusive evidence that stress causes exacerbations. I personally doubt that it causes them alone," said David Mohr, PhD, an associate professor in the department of Psychiatry and Neurology at the University of California, San Francisco.

Dr. Mohr recently conducted a "meta study" of 14 studies on MS and stress, which was published in the March 19, 2004 issue of the *British Medical Journal*. While the data from that study shows an association between stress and exacerbations, Mohr is careful to point out many variables, such as medications, or a viral or bacterial infection. Time is also a major factor, in more ways than one.

When people remember a stressful event, they do so through hindsight. Since memory is often kind, small details tend to get erased and large details can become linked in a way they weren't in reality. "Life is full of stress," Dr. LaRocca said. "You can always find some sort of stressful situation in your life." He pointed out that one of the dilemmas scientists face is that it's "very difficult to go back and retrospectively look at this before people developed MS."

What Is Known About Stress?

Stress initially acts to protect you, releasing chemicals that make your reactions sharper and your mind move faster. Interestingly, the main hormone released during stress, cortisol, is anti-inflammatory, and derivatives of cortisol, such as prednisone, are often used to treat exacerbations. Dr. Mohr said that one possibility is that it's not stress itself that helps cause problems, but rather the resolution of stress, when levels of anti-inflammatory cortisol drop.

Dr. Mohr also points out that exacerbations may originate before stressful events. "Processes are going on that may occur over months, and your body is trying to manage those," he said. "Sometimes those processes get shut down, and sometimes they go on to become full-blown exacerbations." If you are stressed when no exacerbation is developing, then nothing may happen. However, if you are stressed when an exacerbation is developing, Dr. Mohr said, "it may increase the risk a little bit." In other words, stress alone will not cause an exacerbation, but it might be one factor in a complex setoff factors that lead to an exacerbation.

"Saying that stress causes exacerbations is certainly premature," Dr. Mohr said. He is currently enrolling people with MS in the San Francisco Bay and Seattle areas in a study designed to track whether learning stress management techniques can reduce development of new brain lesions or occurrences of new exacerbations. For information about participating, call 800-923-1033 or visitwww.ucsf.edu/bmrc.

Eliminating Stress?

Getting rid of stress is not the same as cutting out French fries. "People with MS have at times been told to quit their jobs to avoid job-related stress," Dr. LaRocca said. "However, people find that if they withdraw from significant life activities, it can actually make their stress worse." Instead, he said, the key is to learn how to deal with stress, not try to escape it.

"I think people have to start by acknowledging that stress is normal in everyday life and that families—with or without MS—have issues that they have to work on and resolve as a family," Dr. Kalb said. She suggests family meetings, family counseling, and individual therapy for figuring out "stress triggers" and managing stress. A stress trigger could be external (noise, disturbing news, caffeine)or internal (depression, anxieties about money, etc.). And no two people are affected the same way by any particular event or thought pattern.

Managing Stress The Healthy Way

After Maggie Staiger was diagnosed, she decided to try hypnosis to help control the pain caused by her MS-related nerve damage. "I was so skeptical because nothing was working," she said, "so why would hypnosis work?" After two sessions, she was convinced—so convinced that she decided to study hypnosis herself and offer hypnosis to other people.

"Through hypnosis you still have all those stresses around you, but you're not responding in a way that is destructive to you," Staiger said. "The stressor of chronic pain is really debilitating, and relieving that stress of always feeling uncomfortable and never getting proper rest was a huge load off me—that made me feel better."

Other people turn to exercise, meditation, prayer groups, or psychotherapy to help with stressful situations, but everyone agrees that whatever you do—or don't do—no one should ever feel guilty about feeling stressed. For better or worse, stress is a normal part of life, and everyone goes through it differently. The person you admire for traveling alone to Tibet may be the person who is barricaded behind the bedroom door during a family picnic.

The relationship between stress and MS is still so tenuous and little understood, that, as Dr. Kalb said, "Until we can explain it, all we can do is encourage people to try to figure out how to handle stresses that are part of their lives"—which, for anyone, can only be a win-win situation.

Chapter 37

Lupus

What is lupus?

Lupus (LOO-puhss) is a chronic, autoimmune (aw-toh-ih-MYOON) disease. It can damage any part of the body (skin, joints, and/or organs inside the body). Chronic means that the signs and symptoms tend to last longer than six weeks and often for many years. In lupus, something goes wrong with your immune system, which is the part of the body that fights off viruses, bacteria, and other germs ("foreign invaders," like the flu). Normally your immune system produces proteins called antibodies that protect the body from these invaders. Autoimmune means your immune system cannot tell the difference between these invaders and your body's healthy tissues ("auto" means "self"). In lupus, your immune system creates autoantibodies (AW-toh-AN-teye-bah-deez), which sometimes attack and destroy healthy tissue. These autoantibodies contribute to inflammation, pain, and damage in various parts of the body.

When people talk about "lupus," they usually mean systemic lupus erythematosus (ur-uh-thee-muh-TOH-suhss), or SLE. This is the most common type of lupus. It is hard to guess how many people in the U.S. have lupus, because the symptoms are so different for every person. Sometimes it is not diagnosed. The Lupus Foundation of America thinks that about 16,000 new cases are reported across the country each year.

Although lupus can affect almost any organ system, the disease, for most people, affects only a few parts of the body. For example, one person with lupus may have swollen knees and fever. Another person may be tired all the time or have kidney trouble. Someone else may have rashes. Over time, more symptoms can develop.

About This Chapter: Information in this chapter is excerpted from "Lupus Fact Sheet," U.S. Department of Health and Human Services, Office on Women's Health (www.womenshealth.gov), June 2011.

Normally, lupus develops slowly, with symptoms that come and go. Women who get lupus most often have symptoms and are diagnosed between the ages of 15 and 45. But the disease also can happen in childhood or later in life.

For some people, lupus is a mild disease. But for others, it may cause severe problems. Even if your lupus symptoms are mild, it is a serious disease that needs constant monitoring and treatment. It can harm your organs and put your life at risk if untreated.

Who gets lupus?

Anyone can get lupus. About nine out of 10 adults with lupus are women ages 15 to 45. African American women are three times more likely to get lupus than white women. Lupus is also more common in Latina, Asian, and Native American women. Men are at a higher risk before puberty and after age 50. Despite an increase in lupus in men in these age groups, two-thirds of the people who have lupus before puberty and after age 50 are women.

African-Americans and Latinos tend to get lupus at a younger age and have more severe symptoms, including kidney problems. African-Americans with lupus have more problems with seizures, strokes, and dangerous swelling of the heart muscle. Latina patients have more heart problems as well. Scientists believe that genes play a role in how lupus affects these ethnic groups.

Apart from genetic factors, lupus can be more severe for people who aren't getting the care they need.

Studies have shown that people with lupus who have a lower household income, lower level of education, or less of a support system tend to do worse with the disease. For some people with lupus, severe symptoms of the disease leave them unable to work, which may result in low income and lack of health insurance. These factors make it hard for a person with lupus to get the right treatment—or sometimes even diagnosis—that they need.

Why is lupus a concern for women?

Lupus is most common in women, especially women in their childbearing years. Having lupus increases your risk of other health problems that are common in women. It can also cause these diseases to occur earlier in life:

- **Heart Disease:** When you have lupus you are at bigger risk of the main type of heart disease, called coronary artery disease (CAD). This is partly because people with lupus have more CAD risk factors, which may include high blood pressure, high cholesterol, and type 2 diabetes.

Lupus Risk Factors And Symptoms

The immune system is designed to attack foreign substances in the body. If you have lupus, something goes wrong with your immune system and it attacks healthy cells and tissues. This can damage many parts of the body such as the:

- Joints
- Kidneys
- Lungs
- Brain
- Skin
- Heart
- Blood vessels

There are many kinds of lupus. The most common type, *systemic lupus erythematosus*, affects many parts of the body.

Who gets lupus?

Anyone can get lupus, but it most often affects women. Lupus is also more common in women of African American, Hispanic, Asian, and Native American descent than in Caucasian women.

What are the symptoms of lupus?

Symptoms of lupus vary, but some of the most common symptoms of lupus are:

- Pain or swelling in joints
- Fever with no known cause
- Chest pain when taking a deep breath
- Pale or purple fingers or toes
- Swelling in legs or around eyes
- Swollen glands
- Muscle pain
- Red rashes, most often on the face
- Hair loss
- Sensitivity to the sun
- Mouth ulcers
- Feeling very tired

Less common symptoms of lupus include:

- Anemia (a decrease in red blood cells)
- Dizzy spells
- Confusion
- Headaches
- Feeling sad
- Seizures

Symptoms may come and go. The times when a person is having symptoms are called flares, which can range from mild to severe. New symptoms may appear at any time.

Source: Excerpted from "What Is Lupus?" National Institute of Arthritis and Musculoskeletal and Skin Diseases (www.niams.nih.gov), October 2009.

- **Osteoporosis (OSS-tee-oh-puh-ROH-suhss):** Women with lupus have more bone loss and broken bones than other women. This might be because some medicines used to treat lupus cause bone loss. The disease itself can also cause bone loss. Also, pain and fatigue can keep women with lupus from exercising. Staying active is important for keeping bones healthy and strong.

- **Kidney Disease:** Many symptoms of lupus come from the swelling of organs in the body. Almost half of all people with lupus develop kidney problems, called lupus nephritis. Kidney problems often begin within the first five years after lupus symptoms start to appear. This is one of the more serious complications of lupus, but there are treatments if problems are caught early. However, it is important to know that kidney inflammation is not painful and you can't feel it. That is why it's important for people with lupus to keep up-to-date with the screenings their doctors recommend.

Pregnancy And Contraception For Women With Lupus

Women with lupus can and do have healthy babies. It is important to involve your health care team during your pregnancy.

Women with lupus who do not wish to become pregnant or who are taking medicine that could be harmful to an unborn baby may want reliable birth control. Recent studies have shown that oral contraceptives (birth control pills) are safe for women with lupus.

Source: Excerpted from "What Is Lupus?" National Institute of Arthritis and Musculoskeletal and Skin Diseases (www.niams.nih.gov), October 2009.

What causes lupus?

The cause of lupus is not known. It's not a disease you can catch from another person. Researchers are looking at these factors:

- Environment (sunlight, stress, smoking, certain medications, and viruses might trigger symptoms in people who are prone to getting lupus)

- Hormones such as estrogen (lupus is more common in women during childbearing years)

- Problems with the immune system

- Genes (Although genes play an important role, they are not the only reason a person will get lupus. Even someone who has one or more of the genes associated with lupus has a small chance of actually getting the disease. Only 10 percent of people with lupus have a parent or sibling who also has it.)

What are flares?

The times when your symptoms worsen and you feel ill are called flares, and they come and go. You may have swelling and rashes one week and no symptoms the next. Sometimes flares occur without clear symptoms and are only seen with laboratory tests. Even if you take medicine for lupus, you may find that some things trigger a flare. For instance, your symptoms may flare after you've been out in the sun or after a hard day at work. Common triggers include:

- Overwork and not enough rest
- Stress
- Being out in the sun or close exposure to fluorescent or halogen light
- Infection
- Injury
- Stopping your lupus medicines
- Certain medications

Is lupus fatal?

Many men and women live long, productive lives with lupus. However, it can be fatal for some people. It depends on the severity of illness, how the body responds to treatments, and other factors. Infections are the leading cause of death in people with lupus. Studies show that people with lupus are living longer lives compared to decades past.

How can my doctor tell if I have lupus?

Lupus can be hard to diagnose. It's often mistaken for other diseases. Many people have lupus for a while before they find out they have it. If you have symptoms, tell your doctor right away. No single test can tell if a person has lupus, but your doctor can find out if you have lupus in other ways, including: medical history, family history, a complete physical exam, blood and urine tests, and a skin or kidney biopsy. Together, this information can provide clues to your disease. It also can help your doctor rule out other diseases that can be confused with lupus.

Should I change my diet because I have lupus?

People with lupus may have to make changes to their diet based on their symptoms, on treatment, and other factors. Ask your doctor if you should eat a special diet because of your lupus.

How is lupus diagnosed?

There is no single test to diagnose lupus. It may take months or years for a doctor to diagnose lupus. Your doctor may use many tools to make a diagnosis:

- Medical history
- Complete exam
- Blood tests
- Skin biopsy (looking at skin samples under a microscope)
- Kidney biopsy (looking at tissue from your kidney under a microscope).

How is lupus treated?

You may need special kinds of doctors to treat the many symptoms of lupus. Your health care team may include:

- A family doctor
- Rheumatologists (treats arthritis and other diseases that cause swelling in the joints)
- Clinical immunologists (treats immune system disorders)
- Nephrologists (treats kidney disease)
- Hematologists (treats blood disorders)
- Dermatologists
- Neurologists (treats problems with the nervous system)
- Cardiologists (treats heart and blood vessel problems)
- Endocrinologists (treats problems related to the glands and hormones)
- Nurses
- Psychologists
- Social workers

Because people with lupus need to avoid the sun, they may lack vitamin D. Your doctor may tell you to take a vitamin for this reason. Herbal supplements have no proven benefit and can cause harm. Talk to your doctor before trying any vitamins or herbal supplements.

Living with lupus can be hard. How can I cope?

Dealing with a long-lasting disease like lupus can be hard on your feelings. Concerns about your health and the effects of your lupus on your work and family life can be stressful. Changes in the way you look and other physical effects of lupus (and the medicines used to treat lupus) can affect your self-esteem.

Your doctor will develop a treatment plan to fit your needs. You and your doctor should review the plan often to be sure it is working. You should report new symptoms to your doctor right away so that treatment can be changed, if needed.

The goals of the treatment plan are to:

- Prevent flares
- Treat flares when they occur
- Reduce organ damage and other problems.

Treatments may include drugs to:

- Reduce swelling and pain
- Prevent or reduce flares
- Help the immune system
- Reduce or prevent damage to joints
- Balance the hormones

In addition to medications for lupus itself, sometimes other medications are needed for problems related to lupus such as high cholesterol, high blood pressure, or infection.

Alternative treatments are those that are not part of standard treatment. No research shows that this kind of treatment works for people with lupus. You should talk to your doctor about alternative treatments.

Source: Excerpted from "What Is Lupus?" National Institute of Arthritis and Musculoskeletal and Skin Diseases (www.niams .nih.gov), October 2009.

Your friends, family, and coworkers might not seem to understand how you feel. At times, you might feel sad or angry. Or, you may feel that you have no control over your life with lupus. But there are things you can do that will help you to cope and to keep a good outlook. Try to:

- **Pace yourself.** People with lupus have less energy and must manage it wisely. Most women with lupus feel much better when they get enough rest and avoid taking on too much at home and at work.

- **Reduce stress.** Exercising with your doctor's okay, finding ways to relax, and staying involved in social activities you enjoy will reduce stress and help you to cope.

- **Get support.** Be open about your feelings and needs with family members and friends. Consider support groups or counseling. They can help you to see that you are not alone.

- **Talk to your doctor.** The symptoms of lupus and some medications can bring on feelings of depression. People with lupus are more likely than others to be depressed and anxious. It is important to tell your doctor about your feelings, so that if it's needed, he or she can treat you for mental health disorders that are more common in people with lupus.

- **Learn about lupus.** People who are well-informed and involved in their own care have less pain, are more active, make fewer visits to the doctor, and feel better about themselves.

What can I do?

It is vital that you take an active role in your treatment. One key to living with lupus is to know about the disease and its impact. Being able to spot the warning signs of a flare can help you prevent the flare or make the symptoms less severe. Many people with lupus have certain symptoms just before a flare, such as: feeling more tired, pain, rash, fever, stomachache, headache, and dizziness. You should see your doctor often, even when symptoms are not severe. These visits will help you and your doctor to:

- Look for changes in symptoms
- Predict and prevent flares
- Change the treatment plan as needed
- Detect side effects of treatment

It is also important to find ways to cope with the stress of having lupus. Exercising and finding ways to relax may make it easier for you to cope. A good support system can also help. A support system may include family, friends, community groups, or doctors. Many people with lupus have found support groups to be very useful. Besides providing support, taking part in a support group can make you feel better about yourself and help you to keep a good outlook.

Learning more about lupus is very important. Studies have shown that patients who are informed and involved in their own care:

- Have less pain
- Make fewer visits to the doctor
- Feel better about themselves
- Remain more active

Source: Excerpted from "What Is Lupus?" National Institute of Arthritis and Musculoskeletal and Skin Diseases (www.niams .nih.gov), October 2009.

Chapter 38

Peptic Ulcers

What is a peptic ulcer?

A peptic ulcer is a sore in the lining of your stomach or duodenum. The duodenum is the first part of your small intestine. A peptic ulcer in the stomach is called a gastric ulcer. One that is in the duodenum is called a duodenal ulcer. A peptic ulcer also may develop just above your stomach in the esophagus, the tube that connects the mouth to the stomach. But most peptic ulcers develop in the stomach or duodenum.

Many people have peptic ulcers. You can have both gastric and duodenal ulcers at the same time and you also can have more than one ulcer in your lifetime.

Peptic ulcers can be treated successfully. Seeing your doctor is the first step.

What causes peptic ulcers?

Most peptic ulcers are caused by:

Helicobacter pylori (*H. pylori*), a germ that causes infection is the most common cause of peptic ulcers. Doctors think *H. pylori* may be spread through unclean food or water or by mouth-to-mouth contact, such as kissing. Even though many people have an *H. pylori* infection, most of them never develop an ulcer.

Use of non-steroidal anti-inflammatory drugs (NSAIDs) is the second most common cause of peptic ulcers. But not everyone who takes NSAIDs gets a peptic ulcer. Ulcers caused by NSAIDs are more often found in people who:

About This Chapter: Information for this chapter is excerpted from "What I Need to Know About Peptic Ulcers," National Institute of Diabetes and Digestive and Kidney Diseases (www.niddk.nih.gov), May 2012.

- Are age 60 or older

- Are female

- Have taken NSAIDs for a long time

- Have had an ulcer before

Other causes of peptic ulcers are rare. One rare cause is Zollinger-Ellison syndrome—a disease that makes the body produce too much stomach acid, which harms the lining of the stomach or duodenum.

Stress or spicy food does not cause peptic ulcers, but either can make ulcer symptoms worse.

Does stress cause ulcers?

No, stress doesn't cause ulcers, but it can make them worse. Most ulcers are caused by a germ called *H. pylori*. Researchers think people might get it through food or water. Most ulcers can be cured by taking a combination of antibiotics and other drugs.

Source: Excerpted from "Stress and Your Health," U.S. Department of Health and Human Services, Office on Women's Health (www.womenshealth.gov), March 2010.

What are the symptoms of peptic ulcers?

A dull or burning pain in your stomach is the most common symptom of peptic ulcers. You may feel the pain anywhere between your belly button and breastbone. The pain often:

- Starts between meals or during the night

- Briefly stops if you eat or take antacids

- Lasts for minutes to hours

- Comes and goes for several days or weeks

Other symptoms of peptic ulcers may include:

- Weight loss

- Poor appetite

- Bloating

- Burping

- Vomiting
- Feeling sick to your stomach

Even if your symptoms are mild, you may have peptic ulcers. You should see your doctor to talk about your symptoms. Peptic ulcers can get worse if they aren't treated.

Call your doctor right away if you have:

- Sudden sharp stomach pain that doesn't go away
- Black or bloody stools
- Bloody vomit or vomit that looks like coffee grounds

These symptoms could be signs an ulcer has:

- Broken a blood vessel
- Gone through, or perforated, your stomach or duodenal wall
- Stopped food from moving from your stomach into the duodenum

These symptoms must be treated quickly. You may need surgery.

How are peptic ulcers diagnosed?

Tell your doctor about your symptoms and which medicines you take. Be sure to mention those you get without a prescription, such as Bayer, Motrin, Advil, or Aleve. These medicines are all NSAIDs.

To see if you have an *H. pylori* infection, your doctor will test your blood, breath, or stool. About half of all people who develop an ulcer from NSAIDs also have an *H. pylori* infection.

Your doctor also may want to look inside your stomach and duodenum by doing an endoscopy or an upper gastrointestinal (GI) series—a type of x ray. Both procedures are painless.

For an endoscopy, you will be given medicine to relax you. Then the doctor will pass an endoscope—a thin, lighted tube with a tiny camera—through your mouth to your stomach and duodenum. Your doctor also may take a small piece of tissue—no bigger than a match head—to look at through a microscope. This process is called a biopsy.

For an upper GI series, you will drink a liquid called barium. The barium will make your stomach and duodenum show up clearly on the x rays.

How are peptic ulcers treated?

If you have peptic ulcers, they can be cured. Depending on what caused your ulcers, your doctor may prescribe one or more of the following medicines:

- A proton pump inhibitor (PPI) or histamine receptor blocker (H2 blocker) to reduce stomach acid and protect the lining of your stomach and duodenum
- One or more antibiotics to kill an *H. pylori* infection
- A medicine that contains bismuth subsalicylate, such as Pepto-Bismol, to coat the ulcers and protect them from stomach acid

These medicines will stop the pain and help heal the ulcers.

If an NSAID caused your peptic ulcers, your doctor may tell you to:

- Stop taking the NSAID
- Reduce how much of the NSAID you take
- Take a PPI or H2 blocker with the NSAID
- Switch to another medicine that won't cause ulcers

You should take:

- Only the medicines your doctor tells you to take
- All medicines exactly as your doctor tells you to, even if your pain stops

Tell your doctor if the medicines make you feel sick or dizzy or cause diarrhea or headaches. Your doctor can change your medicines.

And if you smoke, quit. You also should avoid alcohol. Smoking and drinking alcohol slow the healing of ulcers and can make them worse.

Can antacids or milk help peptic ulcers heal?

Neither antacids—such as Tums—nor milk can heal peptic ulcers, although each may make you feel better briefly. Check with your doctor before taking antacids or drinking milk while your ulcers are healing.

Some of the antibiotics used for *H. pylori* infection may not work as well if you take antacids. And while antacids may make ulcer pain go away for a while, they won't kill the *H. pylori* germ. Only antibiotics can do that.

Many people used to think that drinking milk helped peptic ulcers heal. But doctors know now that while milk may make ulcers feel better briefly, it also increases stomach acid. Too much stomach acid makes ulcers worse.

What if peptic ulcers don't heal?

In many cases, medicines heal ulcers. If an *H. pylori* infection caused your ulcers, you must finish all antibiotics and take any other medicines your doctor prescribes. The infection and ulcers will only heal if you take all medicines as prescribed.

When you have finished your medicines, your doctor will do a breath or stool test to be sure the *H. pylori* infection is gone. Sometimes, the *H. pylori* germ is still there, even after a person has taken all the medicines correctly. If that happens, your doctor will prescribe different antibiotics to get rid of the infection and cure your ulcers.

Rarely, surgery is needed to help ulcers heal. You may need surgery if your ulcers:

- Don't heal
- Keep coming back
- Bleed
- Perforate the stomach or duodenal wall
- Block food from moving out of the stomach

Surgery can:

- Remove the ulcers
- Reduce the amount of acid in your stomach

Can peptic ulcers come back?

Yes. If you smoke or take NSAIDs, your ulcers may come back. If you need to take an NSAID, your doctor may switch you to a different medicine or add medicines to help prevent ulcers.

What can I do to prevent peptic ulcers?

To help prevent ulcers caused by *H. pylori*:

- Wash your hands with soap and water after using the bathroom and before eating.
- Eat food that has been washed well and cooked properly.
- Drink water from a clean, safe source.

To help prevent ulcers caused by NSAIDs:

- Stop using NSAIDs, if possible.

- Take NSAIDs with a meal, if you still need NSAIDs.

- Use a lower dose of NSAIDs.

- Ask your doctor about medicines to protect your stomach and duodenum while taking NSAIDs.

- Ask your doctor about switching to a medicine that won't cause ulcers.

Chapter 39

Chronic Heartburn (GERD)

What is GERD?

Gastroesophageal reflux disease (GERD) is a more serious form of gastroesophageal reflux (GER), which is common. GER occurs when the lower esophageal sphincter (LES) opens spontaneously, for varying periods of time, or does not close properly and stomach contents rise up into the esophagus. GER is also called acid reflux or acid regurgitation, because digestive juices—called acids—rise up with the food. The esophagus is the tube that carries food from the mouth to the stomach. The LES is a ring of muscle at the bottom of the esophagus that acts like a valve between the esophagus and stomach.

When acid reflux occurs, food or fluid can be tasted in the back of the mouth. When refluxed stomach acid touches the lining of the esophagus it may cause a burning sensation in the chest or throat called heartburn or acid indigestion. Occasional GER is common and does not necessarily mean one has GERD. Persistent reflux that occurs more than twice a week is considered GERD, and it can eventually lead to more serious health problems. People of all ages can have GERD.

What are the symptoms of GERD?

The main symptom of GERD in adults is frequent heartburn, also called acid indigestion—burning-type pain in the lower part of the mid-chest, behind the breast bone, and in the mid-abdomen. Most children under 12 years with GERD, and some adults, have GERD without heartburn. Instead, they may experience a dry cough, asthma symptoms, or trouble swallowing.

About This Chapter: The information in this chapter is excerpted from "Heartburn, Gastroesophageal Reflux (GER), and Gastroesophageal Reflux Disease (GERD)," National Institute of Diabetes and Digestive and Kidney Diseases (www.digestive.niddk.nih.gov), April 2012.

What causes GERD?

The reason some people develop GERD is still unclear. However, research shows that in people with GERD, the LES relaxes while the rest of the esophagus is working. Anatomical abnormalities such as a hiatal hernia may also contribute to GERD. A hiatal hernia occurs when the upper part of the stomach and the LES move above the diaphragm, the muscle wall that separates the stomach from the chest. Normally, the diaphragm helps the LES keep acid from rising up into the esophagus. When a hiatal hernia is present, acid reflux can occur more easily. A hiatal hernia can occur in people of any age and is most often a normal finding in otherwise healthy people over age 50. Most of the time, a hiatal hernia produces no symptoms.

Other factors that may contribute to GERD include:

- Obesity

- Pregnancy

- Smoking

Common foods that can worsen reflux symptoms include:

- Citrus fruits

- Chocolate

- Drinks with caffeine or alcohol

- Fatty and fried foods

- Garlic and onions

- Mint flavorings

- Spicy foods

- Tomato-based foods, like spaghetti sauce, salsa, chili, and pizza

Talk with your health care provider if reflux-related symptoms occur regularly and cause you discomfort. Your health care provider may recommend that you eat small, frequent meals and avoid the following foods:

- Sodas that contain caffeine

- Chocolate

- Peppermint

- Spicy foods

- Acidic foods like oranges, tomatoes, and pizza
- Fried and fatty foods

Avoiding food two to three hours before bed may also help.

How is GERD treated?

See your health care provider if you have had symptoms of GERD and have been using antacids or other over-the-counter reflux medications for more than two weeks. Your health care provider may refer you to a gastroenterologist, a doctor who treats diseases of the stomach and intestines. Depending on the severity of your GERD, treatment may involve one or more of the following lifestyle changes, medications, or surgery.

Lifestyle Changes

- If you smoke, stop.
- Avoid foods and beverages that worsen symptoms.
- Lose weight, if needed.
- Eat small, frequent meals.
- Wear loose-fitting clothes.
- Avoid lying down for three hours after a meal.
- Raise the head of your bed six to eight inches by securing wood blocks under the bedposts. Just using extra pillows will not help.

Medications

Your health care provider may recommend over-the-counter antacids or medications that stop acid production or help the muscles that empty your stomach. You can buy many of these medications without a prescription. However, see your health care provider before starting or adding a medication.

- Antacids, such as Alka-Seltzer, Maalox, Mylanta, Rolaids, and Riopan, are usually the first drugs recommended to relieve heartburn and other mild GERD symptoms. Many brands on the market use different combinations of three basic salts—magnesium, calcium, and aluminum—with hydroxide or bicarbonate ions to neutralize the acid in your stomach. Antacids, however, can have side effects. Magnesium salt can lead to diarrhea, and aluminum salt may cause constipation. Aluminum and magnesium salts are often combined in a single product to balance these effects. Calcium carbonate antacids, such as Tums, Titralac, and Alka-2, can also be a supplemental source of calcium. They can cause constipation, as well.

- Foaming agents, such as Gaviscon, work by covering your stomach contents with foam to prevent reflux.

- Histamine receptor blockers (H2 blockers), such as cimetidine (Tagamet HB), famotidine (Pepcid AC), nizatidine (Axid AR), and ranitidine (Zantac 75), decrease acid production. They are available in prescription strength and over-the-counter strength. These drugs provide short-term relief and are effective for about half of those who have GERD symptoms.

- Proton pump inhibitors include omeprazole (Prilosec, Zegerid), lansoprazole (Prevacid), pantoprazole (Protonix), rabeprazole (Aciphex), and esomeprazole (Nexium), which are available by prescription. Prilosec is also available in over-the-counter strength. Proton pump inhibitors are more effective than H2 blockers and can relieve symptoms and heal the esophageal lining in almost everyone who has GERD.

- Prokinetics help strengthen the LES and make the stomach empty faster. This group includes bethanechol (Urecholine) and metoclopramide (Reglan). Metoclopramide also improves muscle action in the digestive tract. Prokinetics have frequent side effects that limit their usefulness— fatigue, sleepiness, depression, anxiety, and problems with physical movement.

Because drugs work in different ways, combinations of medications may help control symptoms. People who get heartburn after eating may take both antacids and H2 blockers. The antacids work first to neutralize the acid in the stomach, and then the H2 blockers act on acid production. By the time the antacid stops working, the H2 blocker will have stopped acid production. Your health care provider is the best source of information about how to use medications for GERD.

What if GERD symptoms persist?

If your symptoms do not improve with lifestyle changes or medications, you may need additional tests.

- Barium swallow radiograph uses x-rays to help spot abnormalities such as a hiatal hernia and other structural or anatomical problems of the esophagus. With this test, you drink a solution and then x-rays are taken. The test will not detect mild irritation, although strictures—narrowing of the esophagus—and ulcers can be observed.

- Upper endoscopy is more accurate than a barium swallow radiograph and may be performed in a hospital or a doctor's office. The doctor may spray your throat to numb it and then, after lightly sedating you, will slide a thin, flexible plastic tube with a light and lens on the end called an endoscope down your throat. Acting as a tiny camera, the endoscope allows the doctor to see the surface of the esophagus and search for abnormalities. If you have had moderate to severe symptoms and this procedure reveals injury to the esophagus, usually no other tests are needed to confirm GERD.

- The doctor also may perform a biopsy. Tiny tweezers, called forceps, are passed through the endoscope and allow the doctor to remove small pieces of tissue from your esophagus. The tissue is then viewed with a microscope to look for damage caused by acid reflux and to rule out other problems if infection or abnormal growths are not found.

- pH monitoring examination involves the doctor either inserting a small tube into the esophagus or clipping a tiny device to the esophagus that will stay there for 24 to 48 hours. While you go about your normal activities, the device measures when, and how much, acid comes up into your esophagus. This test can be useful if combined with a carefully completed diary— recording when, what, and amounts the person eats— which allows the doctor to see correlations between symptoms and reflux episodes. The procedure is sometimes helpful in detecting whether respiratory symptoms, including wheezing and coughing, are triggered by reflux.

A completely accurate diagnostic test for GERD does not exist, and tests have not consistently shown that acid exposure to the lower esophagus directly correlates with damage to the lining.

Surgery

Surgery is an option when medicine and lifestyle changes do not help to manage GERD symptoms. Surgery may also be a reasonable alternative to a lifetime of drugs and discomfort.

Fundoplication is the standard surgical treatment for GERD. Usually a specific type of this procedure, called Nissen fundoplication, is performed. During the Nissen fundoplication, the upper part of the stomach is wrapped around the LES to strengthen the sphincter, prevent acid reflux, and repair a hiatal hernia.

The Nissen fundoplication may be performed using a laparoscope, an instrument that is inserted through tiny incisions in the abdomen. The doctor then uses small instruments that hold a camera to look at the abdomen and pelvis. When performed by experienced surgeons, laparoscopic fundoplication is safe and effective in people of all ages, including infants. The procedure is reported to have the same results as the standard fundoplication, and people can leave the hospital in one to three days and return to work in two to three weeks.

Endoscopic techniques used to treat chronic heartburn include the Bard EndoCinch system, NDO Plicator, and the Stretta system. These techniques require the use of an endoscope to perform the anti-reflux operation. The EndoCinch and NDO Plicator systems involve putting stitches in the LES to create pleats that help strengthen the muscle. The Stretta system uses electrodes to create tiny burns on the LES. When the burns heal, the scar tissue helps toughen the muscle. The long-term effects of these three procedures are unknown.

What are the long-term complications of GERD?

Chronic GERD that is untreated can cause serious complications. Inflammation of the esophagus from refluxed stomach acid can damage the lining and cause bleeding or ulcers—also called esophagitis. Scars from tissue damage can lead to strictures—narrowing of the esophagus—that make swallowing difficult. Some people develop Barrett's esophagus, in which cells in the esophageal lining take on an abnormal shape and color. Over time, the cells can lead to esophageal cancer, which is often fatal. Persons with GERD and its complications should be monitored closely by a physician.

Studies have shown that GERD may worsen or contribute to asthma, chronic cough, and pulmonary fibrosis.

Points To Remember

- Frequent heartburn, also called acid indigestion, is the most common symptom of gastroesophageal reflux disease (GERD) in adults. Anyone experiencing heartburn twice a week or more may have GERD.

- You can have GERD without having heartburn. Your symptoms could include a dry cough, asthma symptoms, or trouble swallowing.

- If you have been using antacids for more than two weeks, it is time to see your health care provider. Most doctors can treat GERD. Your health care provider may refer you to a gastroenterologist, a doctor who treats diseases of the stomach and intestines.

- Health care providers usually recommend lifestyle and dietary changes to relieve symptoms of GERD. Many people with GERD also need medication. Surgery may be considered as a treatment option.

Chapter 40

Irritable Bowel Syndrome

What is irritable bowel syndrome (IBS)?

Irritable bowel syndrome is a functional gastrointestinal (GI) disorder, meaning it is a problem caused by changes in how the GI tract works, but it is not a disease. It is a group of symptoms that occur together. People with a functional GI disorder have frequent symptoms, but the GI tract does not become damaged.

The most common symptoms of IBS are abdominal pain or discomfort, often reported as cramping, along with diarrhea, constipation, or both. In the past, IBS was called colitis, mucous colitis, spastic colon, nervous colon, and spastic bowel. The name was changed to reflect the understanding that the disorder has both physical and mental causes and is not a product of a person's imagination.

IBS is diagnosed when a person has abdominal pain or discomfort at least three times per month for the last three months without other disease or injury that could explain the pain. The pain or discomfort of IBS may occur with a change in stool frequency or consistency or may be relieved by a bowel movement. IBS is often classified into four subtypes based on a person's usual stool consistency. These subtypes are important because they affect the types of treatment that are most likely to improve the person's symptoms.

What is the GI tract?

The GI tract is a series of hollow organs joined in a long, twisting tube from the mouth to the anus. The movement of muscles in the GI tract, along with the release of hormones and

About This Chapter: The information in this chapter is excerpted from "Irritable Bowel Syndrome," National Institute of Diabetes and Digestive and Kidney Diseases (www.digestive.niddk.nih.gov), July 2012.

enzymes, allows for the digestion of food. Organs that make up the GI tract are the mouth, esophagus, stomach, small intestine, large intestine—which includes the appendix, cecum, colon, and rectum—and anus. The intestines are sometimes called the bowel. The last part of the GI tract—called the lower GI tract—consists of the large intestine and anus.

The large intestine absorbs water and any remaining nutrients from partially digested food passed from the small intestine. The large intestine then changes waste from liquid to a solid matter called stool. Stool passes from the colon to the rectum. The rectum is located between the last part of the colon—called the sigmoid colon—and the anus. The rectum stores stool prior to a bowel movement. During a bowel movement, stool moves from the rectum to the anus, the opening through which stool leaves the body.

How common is IBS and who is affected?

Irritable bowel syndrome is estimated to affect three to 20 percent of the population, with most studies ranging from 10 to 15 percent. However, less than one-third of people with the condition see a health care provider for diagnosis. IBS affects about twice as many women as men and is most often found in people younger than 45 years.

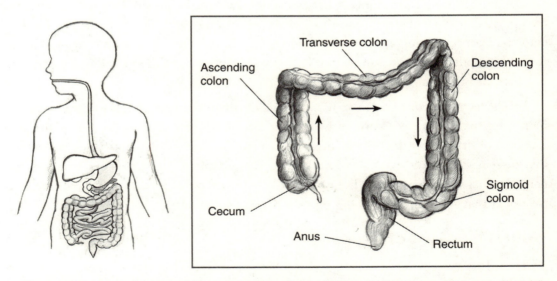

Figure 40.1. The last part of the gastrointestinal (GI) tract, the lower GI tract, consists of the large intestine and the anus. The large intestine absorbs water and remaining nutrients from partially digested food, then changes waste from liquid to a solid matter called stool.

What are the symptoms of IBS?

The symptoms of IBS include abdominal pain or discomfort and changes in bowel habits. To meet the definition of IBS, the pain or discomfort should be associated with two of the following three symptoms: 1) bowel movements occur more or less often than usual; 2) stool appears looser and more watery or harder and more lumpy than usual; and/or 3) improve with a bowel movement. Other symptoms of IBS may include feeling that a bowel movement is incomplete, passing mucus (a clear liquid made by the intestines that coats and protects tissues in the GI tract), and abdominal bloating. Symptoms may often occur after eating a meal. To meet the definition of IBS, symptoms must occur at least three days a month.

What causes IBS?

The causes of IBS are not well understood. Researchers believe a combination of physical and mental health problems can lead to IBS. The possible causes of IBS include the following:

- **Brain-Gut Signal Problems:** Signals between the brain and nerves of the small and large intestines, also called the gut, control how the intestines work.

- **GI Motor Problems:** Normal motility, or movement, may not be present in the colon of a person who has IBS.

- **Hypersensitivity:** People with IBS have a lower pain threshold to stretching of the bowel caused by gas or stool compared with people who do not have IBS.

- **Mental Health Problems:** Mental health, or psychological, problems such as panic disorder, anxiety, depression, and post-traumatic stress disorder are common in people with IBS.

- **Bacterial Gastroenteritis:** Some people who have bacterial gastroenteritis—an infection or irritation of the stomach and intestines caused by bacteria—develop IBS.

- **Small Intestinal Bacterial Overgrowth (SIBO):** Normally, few bacteria live in the small intestine. SIBO is an increase in the number of bacteria or a change in the type of bacteria in the small intestine. These bacteria can produce excess gas and may also cause diarrhea and weight loss.

- **Body Chemicals:** People with IBS have altered levels of neurotransmitters, which are chemicals in the body that transmit nerve signals, and GI hormones, though the role these chemicals play in developing IBS is unclear. Younger women with IBS often have more symptoms during their menstrual periods. Post-menopausal women have fewer symptoms compared with women who are still menstruating. These findings suggest that reproductive hormones can worsen IBS problems.

- **Genetics:** Whether IBS has a genetic cause, meaning it runs in families, is unclear. Studies have shown that IBS is more common in people with family members who have a history of GI problems.

- **Food Sensitivity:** Many people with IBS report that certain foods and beverages can cause symptoms, such as foods rich in carbohydrates, spicy or fatty foods, coffee, and alcohol. However, people with food sensitivity typically do not have clinical signs of food allergy.

How is IBS diagnosed?

To diagnose IBS, a health care provider will conduct a physical exam and take a complete medical history. The medical history will include questions about symptoms, family history of GI disorders, recent infections, medications, and stressful events related to the onset of symptoms. For IBS to be diagnosed, the symptoms must have started at least six months prior and must have occurred at least three days per month for the previous three months. Further testing is not usually needed, though the health care provider may do a blood test to screen for other problems. Additional diagnostic tests may be needed based on the results of the screening blood test and for people who also have signs such as fever, rectal bleeding, weight loss, anemia—or a family history of colon cancer, irritable bowel disease, or celiac disease (immune disease in which people cannot tolerate gluten).

Additional diagnostic tests may include a stool test, lower GI series, and flexible sigmoidoscopy or colonoscopy. Colonoscopy may also be recommended for people who are older than 50 to screen for colon cancer.

How does stress affect IBS?

Stress can stimulate colon spasms in people with IBS. The colon has many nerves that connect it to the brain. These nerves control the normal contractions of the colon and cause abdominal discomfort at stressful times. In people with IBS, the colon can be overly responsive to even slight conflict or stress. Stress makes the mind more aware of the sensations that arise in the colon. IBS symptoms can also increase a person's stress level. Some options for managing stress include:

- Participating in stress reduction and relaxation therapies such as meditation
- Getting counseling and support
- Taking part in regular exercise such as walking or yoga
- Minimizing stressful life situations as much as possible
- Getting enough sleep

Stool Tests: A stool test is the analysis of a sample of stool. The health care provider will give the person a container for catching and storing the stool. The sample is returned to the health care provider or a commercial facility and sent to a lab for analysis. The health care provider may also do a rectal exam, sometimes during the physical exam, to check for blood in the stool. Stool tests can show the presence of parasites or blood.

Lower GI Series: A lower GI series is an x-ray exam that is used to look at the large intestine. The test is performed at a hospital or outpatient center by a radiologist—a doctor who specializes in medical imaging.

Flexible Sigmoidoscopy And Colonoscopy: These tests are similar, but a colonoscopy is used to view the rectum and entire colon, while a flexible sigmoidoscopy is used to view just the rectum and lower colon. These tests are performed at a hospital or outpatient center by a gastroenterologist—a doctor who specializes in digestive diseases.

The gastroenterologist may also perform a biopsy, a procedure that involves taking a piece of intestinal lining for examination with a microscope. You will not feel the biopsy. A pathologist—a doctor who specializes in diagnosing diseases—examines the tissue in a lab.

How is IBS treated?

Though there is no cure for IBS, the symptoms can be treated with a combination of changes in eating, diet, and nutrition; medications; probiotics; and therapies for mental health problems.

Eating, Diet, And Nutrition: Large meals can cause cramping and diarrhea, so eating smaller meals more often, or eating smaller portions, may help IBS symptoms. Eating meals that are low in fat and high in carbohydrates, such as pasta, rice, whole-grain breads and cereals, fruits, and vegetables, may help.

Certain foods and drinks may cause IBS symptoms in some people, such as: foods high in fat; milk products; drinks with alcohol or caffeine; drinks with large amounts of artificial sweeteners; and foods that may cause gas, such as beans and cabbage. People with IBS may want to limit or avoid these foods. Keeping a food diary is a good way to track which foods cause symptoms so they can be excluded from or reduced in the diet.

Dietary fiber may lessen constipation in people with IBS, but it may not help with lowering pain. Fiber helps keep stool soft so it moves smoothly through the colon. The Academy of Nutrition and Dietetics recommends consuming 20 to 35 grams of fiber a day for adults. Fiber may cause gas and trigger symptoms in some people with IBS. Increasing fiber intake by two to three grams per day may help reduce the risk of increased gas and bloating.

Medications: The health care provider will select medications based on the person's symptoms.

- **Fiber Supplements:** Fiber supplements may be recommended to relieve constipation when increasing dietary fiber is ineffective.

- **Laxatives:** Constipation can be treated with laxative medications. Laxatives work in different ways, and a health care provider can provide information about which type is best for each person.

- **Antidiarrheals:** Loperamide has been found to reduce diarrhea in people with IBS, though it does not reduce pain, bloating, or other symptoms.

- **Antispasmodics:** Antispasmodics, such as hyoscine, cimetropium, and pinaverium, help to control colon muscle spasms and reduce abdominal pain.

- **Antidepressants:** Tricyclic antidepressants (TCAs) and selective serotonin reuptake inhibitors (SSRIs) in low doses can help relieve IBS symptoms including abdominal pain.

- **Lubiprostone (Amitiza):** Lubiprostone is prescribed for people who have IBS-C. The medication has been found to improve symptoms of abdominal pain or discomfort, stool consistency, straining, and constipation severity.

The antibiotic rifaximin can reduce abdominal bloating by treating SIBO. But scientists are still debating the use of antibiotics to treat IBS, and more research is needed.

Probiotics: Probiotics are live microorganisms, usually bacteria, that are similar to microorganisms normally found in the GI tract. Studies have found that probiotics, specifically Bifidobacteria and certain probiotic combinations, improve symptoms of IBS when taken in large enough amounts. But more research is needed. Probiotics can be found in dietary supplements, such as capsules, tablets, and powders, and in some foods, such as yogurt. A health care provider can give information about the right kind and right amount of probiotics to take to improve IBS symptoms.

Therapies For Mental Health Problems: The following therapies can help improve IBS symptoms due to mental health problems:

- **Talk Therapy:** Talking with a therapist may reduce stress and improve IBS symptoms. Two types of talk therapy used to treat IBS are cognitive behavioral therapy and psychodynamic, or interpersonal, therapy. Cognitive behavioral therapy focuses on the person's thoughts and actions. Psychodynamic therapy focuses on how emotions affect IBS symptoms. This type of therapy often involves relaxation and stress management techniques.

- **Hypnotherapy:** In hypnotherapy, the therapist uses hypnosis to help the person relax into a trancelike state. This type of therapy may help the person relax the muscles in the colon.

- **Mindfulness Training:** People practicing this type of meditation are taught to focus their attention on sensations occurring at the moment and to avoid worrying about the meaning of those sensations, also called catastrophizing.

Points To Remember

- Irritable bowel syndrome (IBS) is a functional gastrointestinal (GI) disorder, meaning it is a problem caused by changes in how the GI tract works. People with a functional GI disorder have frequent symptoms, but the GI tract does not become damaged.

- IBS is not a disease; it is a group of symptoms that occur together.

- IBS is estimated to affect three to 20 percent of the population, with most studies ranging from 10 to 15 percent.

- The symptoms of IBS include abdominal pain or discomfort and changes in bowel habits. Other symptoms of IBS may include:
  - Diarrhea
  - Constipation
  - Feeling that a bowel movement is incomplete
  - Passing mucus
  - Abdominal bloating

- The causes of IBS are not well understood. Researchers believe a combination of physical and mental health problems can lead to IBS.

- To diagnose IBS, a health care provider will conduct a physical exam and take a complete medical history. The medical history will include questions about symptoms, family history of GI disorders, recent infections, medications, and stressful events related to the onset of symptoms.

- Though there is no cure for IBS, the symptoms can be treated with a combination of the following:
  - Changes in eating, diet, and nutrition
  - Medications
  - Probiotics
  - Therapies for mental health problems

What other conditions are associated with IBS?

People with IBS often suffer from other GI and non-GI conditions. GI conditions such as gastroesophageal reflux disease (GERD) and dyspepsia are more common in people with IBS than the general population. GERD is a condition in which stomach contents flow back up into the esophagus—the organ that connects the mouth to the stomach—because the muscle between the esophagus and the stomach is weak or relaxes when it should not. Dyspepsia, or indigestion, is upper abdominal discomfort that often occurs after eating.

Non-GI conditions often found in people with IBS include:

- Chronic fatigue syndrome (a disorder that causes extreme fatigue, which is tiredness that lasts a long time and limits a person's ability to do ordinary daily activities)

- Chronic pelvic pain

- Temporomandibular joint disorders (problems or symptoms of the chewing muscles and joints that connect the lower jaw to the skull)

- Depression

- Anxiety

- Somatoform disorders (chronic pain or other symptoms with no physical cause that are thought to be due to psychological problems)

Chapter 41

Crohn Disease

Crohn disease is a disease that causes inflammation, or swelling, and irritation of any part of the digestive tract—also called the gastrointestinal (GI) tract. The part most commonly affected is the end part of the small intestine, called the ileum.

The GI tract is a series of hollow organs joined in a long, twisting tube from the mouth to the anus. The movement of muscles in the GI tract, along with the release of hormones and enzymes, allows for the digestion of food.

In Crohn disease, inflammation extends deep into the lining of the affected part of the GI tract. Swelling can cause pain and can make the intestine—also called the bowel—empty frequently, resulting in diarrhea. Chronic (or long-lasting) inflammation may produce scar tissue that builds up inside the intestine to create a stricture. A stricture is a narrowed passageway that can slow the movement of food through the intestine, causing pain or cramps.

Crohn disease is an inflammatory bowel disease (IBD), the general name for diseases that cause inflammation and irritation in the intestines. Crohn disease can be difficult to diagnose because its symptoms are similar to other intestinal disorders, such as ulcerative colitis (and other IBDs) and irritable bowel syndrome. For example, ulcerative colitis and Crohn disease both cause abdominal pain and diarrhea.

Crohn disease may also be called ileitis or enteritis.

About This Chapter: The information in this chapter is excerpted from "Crohn's Disease," National Institute of Diabetes and Digestive and Kidney Diseases (www.digestive.niddk.nih.gov), January 2011.

Who gets Crohn disease?

Crohn disease affects men and women equally and seems to run in some families. People with Crohn disease may have a biological relative—most often a brother or sister—with some form of IBD. Crohn disease occurs in people of all ages, but it most commonly starts in people between the ages of 13 and 30. Men and women who smoke are more likely than nonsmokers to develop Crohn disease. People of Jewish heritage have an increased risk of developing Crohn disease; African Americans have a decreased risk.

What causes Crohn disease?

The cause of Crohn disease is unknown, but researchers believe it is the result of an abnormal reaction by the body's immune system. Normally, the immune system protects people from infection by identifying and destroying bacteria, viruses, or other potentially harmful foreign substances. Researchers believe that in Crohn disease the immune system attacks bacteria, foods, and other substances that are actually harmless or beneficial. During this process, white blood cells accumulate in the lining of the intestines, producing chronic inflammation, which leads to ulcers, or sores, and injury to the intestines.

Researchers have found that high levels of a protein produced by the immune system, called tumor necrosis factor (TNF), are present in people with Crohn disease. However, researchers do not know whether increased levels of TNF and abnormal functioning of the immune system are causes or results of Crohn disease. Research shows that the inflammation seen in the GI tract of people with Crohn disease involves several factors: the genes the person has inherited, the person's immune system, and the environment.

Can stress make Crohn disease worse?

No evidence shows that stress causes Crohn disease. However, people with Crohn disease sometimes feel increased stress in their lives because they live with a chronic illness. Some people with Crohn disease report having a flare up when experiencing a stressful event or situation. For people who find there is a connection between stress level and a worsening of symptoms, using relaxation techniques—such as slow breathing—and taking special care to eat well and get enough sleep may help them feel better. The health care provider may suggest a counselor or support group to help decrease stress for people with Crohn disease.

What are the symptoms of Crohn disease?

The most common symptoms of Crohn disease are abdominal pain, often in the lower right area, and diarrhea. Rectal bleeding, weight loss, and fever may also occur. Bleeding may be serious and persistent, leading to anemia (a condition in which red blood cells are fewer or smaller than normal), which means less oxygen is carried to the body's cells.

The range and severity of symptoms varies.

How is Crohn disease diagnosed?

A doctor will perform a thorough physical exam and schedule a series of tests to diagnose Crohn disease.

- **Blood Tests:** Blood tests can be used to look for anemia caused by bleeding. Blood tests may also uncover a high white blood cell count, which is a sign of inflammation or infection somewhere in the body.

- **Stool Tests:** Stool tests are commonly done to rule out other causes of GI diseases, such as infection. Stool tests can also show if there is bleeding in the intestines.

The following tests are usually performed at a hospital or outpatient center by a gastroenterologist (a doctor who specializes in digestive diseases) or a radiologist (a doctor who specializes in medical imaging).

- **Flexible Sigmoidoscopy And Colonoscopy:** These tests are used to help diagnose Crohn disease and determine how much of the GI tract is affected. Colonoscopy is the most commonly used test to specifically diagnose Crohn disease.

  Colonoscopy is used to view the ileum, rectum, and the entire colon, while flexible sigmoidoscopy is used to view just the lower colon and rectum.

- **Computerized Tomography (CT) Scan:** CT scans use a combination of x rays and computer technology to create three-dimensional (3-D) images.

- **Upper GI Series:** An upper GI series may be done to look at the small intestine.

- **Lower GI Series:** A lower GI series may be done to look at the large intestine.

What are the complications of Crohn disease?

The most common complication of Crohn disease is an intestinal blockage caused by thickening of the intestinal wall because of swelling and scar tissue. Crohn disease may also cause ulcers that tunnel through the affected area into surrounding tissues. The tunnels, called fistulas, are a common complication—especially in the areas around the anus and rectum—and often become infected. Most fistulas can be treated with medication, but some may require surgery. In addition to fistulas, small tears called fissures may develop in the lining of the mucus membrane of the anus. The health care provider may prescribe a topical cream and may suggest soaking the affected area in warm water.

Some Crohn disease complications occur because the diseased area of intestine does not absorb nutrients effectively, resulting in deficiencies of proteins, calories, and vitamins.

People with Crohn disease often have anemia, which can be caused by the disease itself or by iron deficiency. Anemia may make a person feel tired. Children with Crohn disease may fail to grow normally and may have low height for their age.

People with Crohn disease, particularly if they have been treated with steroid medications, may have weakness of their bones called osteoporosis or osteomalacia.

Some people with Crohn disease may have restless legs syndrome—extreme leg discomfort a person feels while sitting or lying down. Some of these problems clear up during treatment for Crohn disease, but some must be treated separately.

Other complications include arthritis, skin problems, inflammation in the eyes or mouth, kidney stones, gallstones, or diseases related to liver function.

What is the treatment for Crohn disease?

Treatment may include medications, surgery, nutrition supplementation, or a combination of these options. The goals of treatment are to control inflammation, correct nutritional deficiencies, and relieve symptoms such as abdominal pain, diarrhea, and rectal bleeding. Treatment for Crohn disease depends on its location, severity, and complications.

Treatment can help control Crohn disease and make recurrences less frequent, but no cure exists. Someone with Crohn disease may need long-lasting medical care and regular doctor visits to monitor the condition. Some people have long periods—sometimes years—of remission when they are free of symptoms, and predicting when a remission may occur or when symptoms will return is not possible. This changing pattern of the disease makes it difficult to be certain a treatment has helped.

Despite possible hospitalizations and the need to take medication for long periods of time, most people with Crohn disease have full lives—balancing families, careers, and activities.

Medications: Medications for Crohn disease include anti-inflammatory agents, corticosteroids, immunosuppressive medications, biological therapies, antibiotics, and antidiarrheal medications and fluid replacements:

- **Anti-Inflammation Medications:** Most people are first treated with medications containing mesalamine, a substance that helps control inflammation. Sulfasalazine is the most commonly used of these medications. People who do not benefit from sulfasalazine or who cannot tolerate it may be put on other mesalamine-containing medications, known as 5-aminosalicylic acid (5-ASA) agents, such as Asacol, Dipentum, or Pentasa. Possible side effects of mesalamine-containing medications include nausea, vomiting, heartburn, diarrhea, and headache.

- **Cortisone Or Steroids:** These medications, also called corticosteroids, are effective at reducing inflammation. Prednisone and budesonide are generic names of two corticosteroids. During the earliest stages of Crohn disease, when symptoms are at their worst, corticosteroids are usually prescribed in a large dose. The dosage is then gradually lowered once symptoms are controlled. Corticosteroids can cause serious side effects, including greater susceptibility to infection and osteoporosis, or weakening of the bones.

- **Immune System Suppressors:** Medications that suppress the immune system—called immunosuppressive medications—are also used to treat Crohn disease. The most commonly prescribed medications are 6-mercaptopurine and azathioprine. Immunosuppressive medications work by blocking the immune reaction that contributes to inflammation. These medications may cause side effects such as nausea, vomiting, and diarrhea and may lower a person's resistance to infection. Some people are treated with a combination of corticosteroids and immunosuppressive medications. Some studies suggest that immunosuppressive medications may enhance the effectiveness of corticosteroids.

- **Biological Therapies:** Biological therapies are medications given by an injection in the vein, infliximab (Remicade), or an injection in the skin, adalimumab (HUMIRA). Biological therapies bind to TNF substances to block the body's inflammation response. The U.S. Food and Drug Administration approved these medications for the treatment of moderate to severe Crohn disease that does not respond to standard therapies—mesalamine substances, corticosteroids, immunosuppressive medications—and for the treatment of open, draining fistulas. Some studies suggest that biological therapies may enhance the effectiveness of immunosuppressive medications.

- **Antibiotics:** Antibiotics are used to treat bacterial overgrowth in the small intestine caused by stricture, fistulas, or surgery. For this common problem, the doctor may prescribe one or more of the following antibiotics: ampicillin, sulfonamide, cephalosporin, tetracycline, or metronidazole.

- **Antidiarrheal Medications And Fluid Replacements:** Diarrhea and abdominal cramps are often relieved when the inflammation subsides, but additional medication may be needed. Anti-diarrheal medications include diphenoxylate, loperamide, and codeine. People with diarrhea should drink plenty of fluids to prevent dehydration. If diarrhea does not improve, the person should see the doctor promptly for possible treatment with intravenous fluids.

Surgery: About two-thirds of people with Crohn disease will require surgery at some point in their lives. Surgery becomes necessary to relieve symptoms that do not respond to medical therapy or to correct complications such as intestinal blockage, perforation, bleeding, or abscess—a painful, swollen, pus-filled area caused by infection. Surgery to remove part of the intestine can help people with Crohn disease, but it does not eliminate the disease. People with Crohn disease commonly need more than one operation because inflammation tends to return to the area next to where the diseased intestine was removed.

Because Crohn disease often recurs after surgery, people considering surgery should carefully weigh its benefits and risks compared with other treatments. People faced with this decision should get information from health care providers who routinely work with GI patients, including those who have had intestinal surgery. Patient advocacy organizations can suggest support groups and other information resources.

Nutrition Supplementation: The health care provider may recommend nutritional supplements, especially for children whose growth has been slowed. Special high-calorie liquid formulas are sometimes used. A small number of people may receive nutrition intravenously for a brief time through a small tube inserted into an arm vein. This procedure can help people who need extra nutrition temporarily, such as those whose intestines need to rest, or those whose intestines cannot absorb enough nutrition from food.

The doctor may prescribe calcium, vitamin D, and other medications to prevent or treat osteoporosis for patients taking corticosteroids. People should take vitamin supplements only after talking with their doctor.

Eating, Diet, And Nutrition: No special diet has been proven effective for preventing or treating Crohn disease, but it is important that people who have Crohn disease follow a nutritious diet and avoid any foods that seem to worsen symptoms. People with Crohn disease often experience a decrease in appetite, which can affect their ability to receive the daily nutrition needed for good health and healing. In addition, Crohn disease is associated with diarrhea and poor absorption of necessary nutrients. Foods do not cause Crohn disease, but foods such as bulky grains, hot spices, alcohol, and milk products may increase diarrhea and cramping. The health care provider may refer a person with Crohn disease to a dietitian for guidance about meal planning.

Can smoking make Crohn disease worse?

Studies have shown that people with Crohn disease who smoke may have more severe symptoms and increased complications of the disease, along with a need for higher doses of steroids and other medications. People with Crohn disease who smoke are also more likely to need surgery. Quitting smoking can greatly improve the course of Crohn disease and help reduce the risk of complications and flare ups. A health care provider can assist people in finding a smoking cessation specialist.

Is pregnancy safe for women with Crohn disease?

Women with Crohn disease can become pregnant and have a baby. Even so, women with Crohn disease should talk with their health care provider before getting pregnant. Most children born to women with Crohn disease are not affected by the condition.

Points To Remember

- Crohn disease is a disease that causes inflammation, or swelling, and irritation of any part of the digestive tract—also called the gastrointestinal (GI) tract.
- Crohn disease affects men and women equally and seems to run in some families.
- The cause of Crohn disease is unknown, but researchers believe it is the result of an abnormal reaction by the immune system.
- The most common symptoms of Crohn disease are abdominal pain and diarrhea.
- A doctor can diagnose Crohn disease by performing a physical exam, blood and stool tests, and imaging tests such as a CT scan, upper GI series, lower GI series, flexible sigmoidoscopy, and colonoscopy.
- The most common complication of Crohn disease is an intestinal blockage caused by thickening of the intestinal wall because of swelling and scar tissue.
- Doctors treat Crohn disease with medications, surgery, nutrition supplementation, or a combination of these options.
- No special diet has been proven effective for preventing or treating Crohn disease, but it is important that people who have Crohn disease follow a nutritious diet and avoid any foods that seem to worsen symptoms.
- Some people with Crohn disease report having a flare up when experiencing a stressful event or situation. The health care provider may suggest a counselor or support group to help decrease stress for people with Crohn disease.
- Women with Crohn disease can become pregnant and have a baby. Even so, women with Crohn disease should talk with their health care provider before getting pregnant.

Chapter 42

Ulcerative Colitis

Ulcerative colitis (UC) is a chronic, or long-lasting, disease that causes inflammation and sores, called ulcers, in the inner lining of the large intestine, which includes the colon and the rectum—the end part of the colon.

UC is one of the two main forms of chronic inflammatory disease of the gastrointestinal tract, called inflammatory bowel disease (IBD). The other form is called Crohn disease.

Normally, the large intestine absorbs water from stool and changes it from a liquid to a solid. In UC, the inflammation causes loss of the lining of the colon, leading to bleeding, production of pus, diarrhea, and abdominal discomfort.

What causes UC?

The cause of UC is unknown though theories exist. People with UC have abnormalities of the immune system, but whether these problems are a cause or a result of the disease is still unclear. The immune system protects people from infection by identifying and destroying bacteria, viruses, and other potentially harmful foreign substances. With UC, the body's immune system is believed to react abnormally to bacteria in the digestive tract. UC sometimes runs in families and research studies have shown that certain gene abnormalities are found more often in people with UC.

UC is not caused by emotional distress, but the stress of living with UC may contribute to a worsening of symptoms. In addition, while sensitivity to certain foods or food products does not cause UC, it may trigger symptoms in some people.

About This Chapter: The information in this chapter is excerpted from "Ulcerative Colitis," National Institute of Diabetes and Digestive and Kidney Diseases (www.digestive.niddk.nih.gov), November 2011.

What are the symptoms of UC?

The most common symptoms of UC are abdominal discomfort and blood or pus in diarrhea. Other symptoms include:

- Anemia

- Fatigue

- Fever

- Nausea

- Weight loss

- Loss of appetite

- Rectal bleeding

- Loss of body fluids and nutrients

- Skin lesions

- Growth failure in children

Most people diagnosed with UC have mild to moderate symptoms. About 10 percent have severe symptoms such as frequent fevers, bloody diarrhea, nausea, and severe abdominal cramps. UC can also cause problems such as joint pain, eye irritation, kidney stones, liver disease, and osteoporosis.

Who develops UC?

While UC can occur in people of any age, it usually develops between the ages of 15 and 30 and less frequently between the ages of 60 and 80. The disease affects men and women equally. People with a family member or first-degree relative with an IBD are at higher risk for developing UC, as are Caucasians and people of Jewish descent.

How is UC diagnosed?

Ulcerative colitis can be difficult to diagnose because its symptoms are similar to those of other intestinal disorders and to Crohn disease. Crohn disease differs from UC in that Crohn disease causes inflammation deeper within the intestinal wall and can occur in other parts of the digestive system, including the small intestine, mouth, esophagus, and stomach.

People with suspected UC may be referred to a gastroenterologist, also called a gastroenterological specialist, a doctor who specializes in digestive diseases. A physical exam and medical history are usually the first steps in diagnosing UC, followed by one or more tests and procedures:

- **Blood Tests:** The blood test can show a high white blood cell (WBC) count, which is a sign of inflammation somewhere in the body. Blood tests can also detect anemia, which could be caused by bleeding in the colon or rectum.

- **Stool Test:** Stool tests can show WBCs, which indicate UC or another IBD. The sample also allows doctors to detect bleeding or infection in the colon or rectum caused by bacteria, a virus, or parasites.

- **Flexible Sigmoidoscopy And Colonoscopy:** These tests are the most accurate methods for diagnosing UC and ruling out other possible conditions, such as Crohn disease, diverticular disease, or cancer. The tests are similar, but colonoscopy is used to look inside the rectum and entire colon, while flexible sigmoidoscopy is used to look inside the rectum and lower colon.

- **Computerized Tomography (CT) Scan And Barium Enema X-Ray:** A CT scan uses a combination of x-rays and computer technology to create three-dimensional (3-D) images. These tests can show physical abnormalities and are sometimes used to diagnose UC.

How is UC treated?

Treatment for UC depends on the severity of the disease and its symptoms. Each person experiences UC differently, so treatment is adjusted for each individual.

Medication Therapy: While no medication cures UC, many can reduce symptoms. The goals of medication therapy are to induce and maintain remission—periods when the symptoms go away for months or even years—and to improve quality of life. Many people with UC require medication therapy indefinitely, unless they have their colon and rectum surgically removed.

The type of medication prescribed depends on the severity of the UC.

- **Aminosalicylates:** These medications contain 5-aminosalicyclic acid (5-ASA) and help control inflammation.

- **Corticosteroids:** Prednisone, methylprednisone, and hydrocortisone are corticosteroids, which help reduce inflammation. They are used for people with more severe symptoms and people who do not respond to 5-ASAs. Corticosteroids are also known as steroids. Side effects include weight gain, acne, facial hair, hypertension, diabetes, mood swings, bone mass loss, and an increased risk of infection. Because of harsh side effects, steroids are not recommended for long-term use. Steroids are usually prescribed for short-term use and then stopped once inflammation is under control. The other UC medications are used for long-term symptom management.

- **Immunomodulators:** Azathioprine (Imuran, Azasan), 6-mercaptopurine (6-MP) (Purinethol), and cyclosporine (Neoral, Sandimmun, Sandimmune) are immunomodulators, which suppress the immune system. These medications are prescribed for people who do not respond to 5-ASAs. People taking these medications are monitored for complications including nausea, vomiting, fatigue, pancreatitis, hepatitis, a reduced WBC count, and an increased risk of infection.

- **Infliximab:** An anti-tumor necrosis factor (anti-TNF) agent, infliximab (Remicade), is prescribed to treat people who do not respond to the other UC medications or who cannot take 5-ASAs. People taking infliximab should also take immunomodulators to avoid allergic reactions. Infliximab targets a protein called TNF that causes inflammation in the intestinal tract. Side effects may include toxicity and increased risk of infections, particularly tuberculosis.

Other medications may be prescribed to decrease emotional stress or to relieve pain, reduce diarrhea, or stop infection.

Hospitalization: Sometimes UC symptoms are severe enough that a person must be hospitalized. For example, a person may have severe bleeding or diarrhea that causes dehydration. In such cases, health care providers will use intravenous fluids to treat diarrhea and loss of blood, fluids, and mineral salts. People with severe symptoms may need a special diet, tube feeding, medications, or surgery.

Surgery: About 10 to 40 percent of people with UC eventually need a proctocolectomy (a surgery to remove the rectum and part, or all of, the colon). Surgery is sometimes recommended if medical treatment fails or if the side effects of corticosteroids or other medications threaten a person's health. Other times surgery is performed because of massive bleeding, severe illness, colon rupture, or cancer risk. Surgery is performed at a hospital by a surgeon; anesthesia will be used. Most people need to remain in the hospital for one to two weeks, and full recovery can take four to six weeks.

A proctocolectomy is followed by one of the following operations:

- **Ileoanal Pouch Anastomosis:** Also called "pouch surgery," this surgery makes it possible for people with UC to have normal bowel movements, because it preserves part of the anus. Waste is stored in the pouch and passes through the anus in the usual manner. Bowel movements may be more frequent and watery than before the procedure. Inflammation of the pouch, called pouchitis, is a possible complication and can lead to symptoms such as increased diarrhea, rectal bleeding, and loss of bowel control. Pouch surgery is the first type of surgery considered for UC because it avoids a long-term ileostomy.

- **Ileostomy:** This operation attaches the ileum to an opening made in the abdomen, called a stoma. An ostomy pouch is then attached to the stoma and worn outside the body to collect stool. The pouch needs to be emptied several times a day. An ileostomy performed for UC is usually permanent.

The type of surgery recommended will be based on the severity of the disease and the person's needs, expectations, and lifestyle. People faced with this decision should get as much information as possible. Patient advocacy organizations can provide information about support groups and other resources.

Eating, Diet, And Nutrition: Dietary changes may help reduce UC symptoms. A recommended diet will depend on the person's symptoms, medications, and reactions to food. General dietary tips that may alleviate symptoms include:

- Eating smaller meals more often

- Avoiding carbonated drinks

- Eating bland foods

- Avoiding high-fiber foods such as corn and nuts

For people with UC who do not absorb enough nutrients, vitamin and nutritional supplements may be recommended.

Is colon cancer a concern with UC?

People with UC have an increased risk of colon cancer when the entire colon is affected for a long period of time. For example, if only the lower colon and rectum are involved, the risk of cancer is no higher than that of a person without UC. But if the entire colon is involved, the risk of cancer is higher than the normal rate. The risk of colon cancer also rises after having UC for eight to 10 years and continues to increase over time. Effective maintenance of remission by treatment of UC may reduce the risk of colon cancer. Surgical removal of the colon eliminates the risk of colon cancer.

With UC, precancerous changes (called dysplasia) sometimes occur in the cells lining the colon. People with dysplasia are at increased risk of developing colon cancer. Doctors look for signs of dysplasia when performing a colonoscopy or flexible sigmoidoscopy and when examining tissue removed during these procedures.

According to the U.S. Preventive Services Task Force guidelines for colon cancer screening, people who have had IBD throughout the colon for at least eight years and those who have had IBD in only the left side of the colon for 12 to 15 years should have a colonoscopy with biopsies every one to two years to check for dysplasia. Such screening has not been proven to reduce the risk of colon cancer, but it may help identify cancer early and improve prognosis.

Points To Remember

- Ulcerative colitis (UC) is a chronic, or long-lasting, disease that causes inflammation and sores, called ulcers, in the inner lining of the colon and rectum.
- Ulcerative colitis is one of the two main forms of chronic inflammatory disease of the gastrointestinal tract, called inflammatory bowel disease (IBD).
- The most common symptoms of UC are abdominal discomfort and bloody diarrhea.
- UC is not caused by emotional distress, but the stress of living with UC may contribute to a worsening of symptoms.
- Flexible sigmoidoscopy and colonoscopy are the most accurate methods for diagnosing UC and ruling out other possible conditions, such as Crohn disease, diverticular disease, or cancer.
- Treatment for UC depends on the severity of the disease and its symptoms. Each person experiences UC differently, so treatment is adjusted for each individual.
- Most people with UC never develop colon cancer, but two factors can increase the risk: the duration of the disease and how much of the colon is affected.

Chapter 43

Eczema

The Impact Of Stress On Eczema

The impact of stress has long been seen as a contributing factor for those who battle with atopic eczema but the correlation between the two has never been categorically and universally proven.

Stress is one of a number of lifestyle influences that appear to make perfect sense when looking at what triggers a flare-up of eczema or make an existing problem worse. I'm also comfortable to put to rest any preconception that stress is solely a female-only domain. The issue has always been trying to pinpoint whether the stress causes the eczema or vice versa.

There's been a degree of research into this area in various countries. Most recently, a Swedish study into lifestyle factors and hand eczema concluded that there was a correlation and it was more common among individuals who reported high stress levels.

Another study at the Yonsei University College of Medicine in Seoul compared the degree of psychological stress in those with atopic dermatitis and those without. The Korean study concluded that anxiety may be associated with the start of the eczema itch (pruritus).

Details of both of these studies were sourced from PubMed—an exhaustive online resource on all manner of health trials and studies worldwide including eczema. You can read the "abstract" or summary of a study for free but there's often a cost to read the full article—which isn't usually necessary to get a flavor of what was the final scientific conclusion. It's worth

About This Chapter: "The Impact of Stress on Eczema," by John Fuller, a freelance journalist with severe atopic eczema. Reprinted with permission from the December 2011 issue of *Exchange*, a publication of the National Eczema Society, www.eczema.org. The National Eczema Society is registered as a charity with the charity commission of England and Wales under No 1009671.

noting that the content isn't written with the average eczema patient in mind but for an overview of eczema research, it's as good as any.

Neither of the outcomes in Sweden or Korea will be earth-shattering news for patients with eczema who suspected as much all along. Thankfully, the absence of conclusive scientific proof needn't stop patients being proactive around their own eczema by controlling certain aspects that could be helpful in coping with stress.

One of the most disturbing and difficult things with eczema is the feeling of helplessness when the condition gets to a point where it controls you rather than the other way around. Obviously, avoiding stress is far easier said than done, particularly as it manifests itself in a myriad of ways, such as issues with relationships with friends and family, employment, and financial worries.

Spotting The Triggers

So, what can those with eczema do to manage their stress more effectively? Spotting the early signs of stress and acting quickly—as you would with a flare-up of eczema itself—is likely to be helpful but not always realistic.

It's often not possible to avoid stress completely but keeping a stress diary for a few weeks to identify the links between stress and eczema—what you were doing, how you felt, and how your eczema responded—might give you some pointers.

Admittedly, this won't be for everyone but it could be worth trying once to gauge any noticeable benefits. As with so much about eczema, the individual nature of the impact of stress on a person's eczema is going to vary enormously. Some people find stress triggers their eczema immediately while others experience a delay so it can be several days before the impact on their skin is felt.

There can be no greater expert than the person with the eczema, or their caretaker, to gauge to what degree stress influences their condition. Frustratingly, there is no one-size-fits-all answer as regards to stress. Finding something that works for you is likely to take some investment but it might prove fruitful.

It's also worth reiterating that it's highly unlikely that eczema is triggered by a single factor alone. So while understanding stress and trying to manage it is definitely an approach to take, it's one of a number of areas to keep thinking about. Keeping on top of your ongoing treatment and seeing a general practitioner (GP) or dermatologist are not to be forfeited in favor of more yoga!

There's no escaping the fact that just having eczema is inherently stressful from the outset. By its very nature, whereby the person with eczema causes the damage to the skin, there can be a degree of guilt or emotional stress as part of the condition. Therefore, having the support and understanding of friends and family is hugely significant.

Talking through worries rather than letting them build might defuse a particular anxiety—it won't rid you of eczema but it might enable you to feel up to tackling it head-on once more. If the eczema is out of control—or having a negative impact on sleep, work, or relationships—map out a plan of action to get back that control.

That might be through organizing a dermatology referral or researching new treatments. No one should have to put up with eczema that's not being managed effectively, and there's always something else to be done to try to improve the tough scenario of living with the condition.

Learning To Relax

If trying to identify what aspects in life are causing you stress and perhaps contributing to your eczema, learning to relax is the next step.

Everyone relaxes in different ways and just being told to "relax" is not likely to magically reap benefits. However, embracing the philosophy through some of the available relaxation methods—like deep breathing techniques, reading, relaxing in a bath, indulging in a hobby, or doing some exercise—might prove beneficial.

None of these sound particularly revolutionary, but coping with a debilitating skin condition is attritional, alongside all the other challenges life throws up. Making time to relax or relieve stress—however that works for you—is important and could be built into a daily routine.

Aside from some of the more conventional methods mentioned here, everything from aromatherapy, massage, reflexology, yoga, meditation, or hypnosis offers ways to relax, particularly as an aid to sleep.

Habit Scratching

The relevance of stress to eczema is perhaps most applicable when looking at habit scratching. Given that eczema is a long-term chronic condition, and the itch and scratching is part and parcel of that, the habit of scratching can become so engrained that doing it becomes second nature—whether or not the skin is actually itchy.

Reacting to a stressful situation, and perhaps not coping with it very well, can result in a bout of fierce scratching as a coping mechanism or nervous reaction. What might have started purely because of a stressful scenario becomes part of the dreaded "itch-scratch" cycle and results in a flare-up.

Breaking this cycle and the resulting or accompanying stress is never easy, but is easiest when done early. The eczema and the stress are interwoven and—at the start of a period of itchiness—the absolutely last thing that will come naturally is practicing relaxed breathing or wanting to relax in a bath.

At these distressing times, distraction before relaxation is often the best weapon against a severe outbreak of scratching. Physically moving into a new room can jolt a person out of that initial risk of staying in situ and doing real damage to the skin.

The start of any eczema flare lends itself to a snowball effect in worsening symptoms and the accompanying stress plays a part. It would take someone with unheard-of levels of self-discipline to react with clinical efficiency to each bout of itchiness.

Personally, a combination of immediate ice packs to cool the skin and something visual to deflect my honed attention away from my skin—like a computer game or film—can sometimes be enough. The key is to act immediately and decisively. There is a window of opportunity at the start of a flare, but it isn't open for long. Stress also lies in the unknown—not knowing how serious a flare will be, whether it will be controlled and the resulting ripple effect it might have on life.

Having eczema or caring for someone with eczema can involve some detective work. Identifying triggers and environmental factors, such as certain times of day or even specific areas of the house where scratching takes place, is all information to gather. Getting a small insight into any of these clues will help to identify scenarios to try to avoid.

Ultimately, whether stress fuels the eczema or the other way round, there are always options open to help us all deal positively with stress—both in the context of our own eczema and with life as a whole.

Does stress cause acne?

Stress doesn't cause acne, but research suggests that for people who have acne, stress can make it worse.

Source: Excerpted from "Questions and Answers about Acne," National Institute of Arthritis and Musculoskeletal and Skin Diseases (NIAMS), October 2012; full text available online at http://www.niams.nih.gov/health_info/acne.

Chapter 44

Hair Loss

Baldness or hair loss is usually something only adults need to worry about. But in a few cases, teens lose their hair, too—and it may be a sign that something's going on.

Hair loss during adolescence can mean a person may be sick or just not eating right. Some medications or medical treatments, like chemotherapy treatment for cancer, also cause hair loss. People can even lose their hair if they wear a hairstyle that pulls on the hair for a long time, such as braids.

Losing hair can be stressful during a time when you're already concerned about appearance. Most of the time, hair loss during the teen years is temporary. With temporary hair loss, the hair usually grows back after the problem that causes it is corrected.

Hair Basics

Hair is made of a type of protein called keratin. A single hair consists of a hair shaft (the part that shows), a root below the skin, and a follicle, from which the hair root grows. At the lower end of the follicle is the hair bulb, where the hair's color pigment, or melanin, is produced.

Most people lose about 50 to 100 head hairs a day. These hairs are replaced—they grow back in the same follicle on your head. This amount of hair loss is totally normal and no cause for worry. If you're losing more than that, though, something might be wrong.

About This Chapter: "Hair Loss," October, 2011, reprinted with permission from www.kidshealth.org. This information was provided by KidsHealth®, one of the largest resources online for medically reviewed health information written for parents, kids, and teens. For more articles like this, visit www.KidsHealth.org or www .TeensHealth.org. Copyright © 1995–2012 The Nemours Foundation. All rights reserved.

If you have hair loss and don't know what's causing it, talk to your doctor. A doctor can determine why the hair is falling out and suggest a treatment that will correct the underlying problem, if necessary.

What Causes Hair Loss?

Here are some of the things that can cause hair loss in teens:

- **Illnesses Or Medical Conditions:** Endocrine (hormonal) conditions, such as uncontrolled diabetes or thyroid disease, can interfere with hair production and cause hair loss. People with lupus can also lose hair. The hormone imbalance that occurs in polycystic ovary syndrome can cause hair loss in teen girls as well as adult women.

- **Medications:** Some medications that have hair loss as a side effect may be prescribed for teens. These include acne medicines like isotretinoin, and lithium, which is used to treat bipolar disorder. Diet pills that contain amphetamines also can cause hair loss. Chemotherapy drugs for cancer are probably the most well-known medications that cause hair loss

- **Alopecia Areata:** This skin disease causes hair loss on the scalp and sometimes elsewhere on the body. It affects 1.7% of the population, including more than five million people in the United States. Alopecia areata (pronounced: al-uh-pee-shuh air-ee-ah-tuh) is thought to be an autoimmune disease, in which the hair follicles are damaged by a person's own immune system. (In autoimmune diseases, the immune system mistakenly attacks healthy cells, tissues, and organs in a person's body.)

  Alopecia areata usually starts as one or more small, round bald patches on the scalp. These can get bigger, and in a small number of cases, can progress to total hair loss. Both guys and girls can get it, and it often begins in childhood. The hair usually grows back within a year, but not always. Sometimes people with alopecia areata lose their hair again.

- **Trichotillomania:** Trichotillomania (pronounced: trik-o-til-uh-may-nee-uh) is a psychological disorder in which people repeatedly pull their hair out, often leaving bald patches. It results in areas of baldness and damaged hairs of different lengths. People with trichotillomania usually need professional help from a therapist or other mental health professional before they are able to stop pulling their hair out.

- **Hair Treatments And Styling:** Having your hair chemically treated, such as getting your hair colored, bleached, straightened, or permed, and applying heat to hair (like using a hot iron or hot blow drying) can cause damage that may make the hair break off or fall out temporarily. Another type of baldness that results from hair styling actually can be permanent: Wearing hair pulled so tightly that it places tension on the scalp can result in a condition called traction alopecia. Traction alopecia can be permanent if the style is worn for a long enough time that it damages the hair follicles.

- **Poor Nutrition:** Poor eating can contribute to hair loss. This is why some people with eating disorders like anorexia and bulimia lose their hair: The body isn't getting enough protein, vitamins, and minerals to sustain hair growth. Some teens who are vegetarians also lose their hair if they don't get enough protein from non-meat sources. And some athletes are at higher risk for hair loss because they may be more likely to develop iron-deficiency anemia.

- **Disruption Of The Hair Growth Cycle:** Some major events can alter the hair's growth cycle temporarily. For example, delivering a baby, having surgery, going through a traumatic event, or having a serious illness or high fever can temporarily cause shedding of large amounts of hair. Because the hair we see on our heads has actually taken months to grow, a person might not notice any disruption of the hair growth cycle until months after the event that caused it. This type of hair loss corrects itself.

- **Androgenetic Alopecia:** Among adults, the most common cause of hair loss is androgenetic (pronounced: an-druh-juh-neh-tik) alopecia, sometimes called male- or female-pattern baldness. This condition is caused by a combination of factors, including hormones called androgens and genetics. Sometimes, the hair loss can start as early as the mid-teen years. It also can occur in people who take steroids like testosterone to build their bodies.

What Can Doctors Do?

If you see a doctor about hair loss, he or she will ask questions about your health and family health (called a medical history) and check your scalp. In some cases, the doctor might take hair samples and test for certain medical conditions that can cause hair loss.

If medication is causing hair loss, ask the doctor if you can take a different drug. If your hair loss is due to an endocrine condition, like diabetes or thyroid disease or female-pattern baldness, proper treatment and control of the underlying disorder is important to reduce or prevent hair loss.

If your doctor recommends it, a product like minoxidil that can increase hair growth in male-pattern baldness also might be helpful. Alopecia areata can be helped by treatment with corticosteroids. If nutritional deficiencies are found to be causing your hair loss, the doctor might refer you to a dietitian or other nutrition expert.

Catastrophic Hair Loss

Hair loss can be the first outward sign that a person is sick, so it may feel scary. Teens who have cancer and lose their hair because of chemotherapy treatments (especially girls) might go through a difficult time.

It can help to feel like you have some control over your appearance when you're losing your hair. When getting chemotherapy, some people like to cut their hair or shave their heads before the hair falls out. Some even take the hair they cut off and have it made into a wig.

Many options can help disguise hair loss—such as wearing wigs, hair wraps, hats, and baseball caps. For most teens who lose their hair, the hair does return—including after chemotherapy.

Taking Care Of Your Hair

Eating a balanced, healthy diet is important for a lot of reasons, and it really benefits your hair.

If you're losing hair, some doctors recommend using baby shampoo, shampooing no more than once a day, and lathering gently. Don't rub your hair too vigorously with a towel, either. Many hair experts suggest putting away the blow dryer and air drying your hair instead. If you can't live without your blow dryer, try using it on a low-heat setting.

Style your hair when it's dry or damp. Styling your hair while it's wet can cause it to stretch and break. And try to avoid teasing your hair, which can cause damage. Finally, be careful when using chemicals—such as straighteners or color—on your hair, and avoid frequent use of chemical treatments.

Part Five
Stress Management

Chapter 45

Talk To Your Parents Or Other Adults

You probably talk to friends way more than you talk to your parents. That's natural. Even if you and your parents have a great relationship, you want to find your own path and make your own choices.

Still, most of us want a parent's help, advice, and support at times. But talking to the adults in your life can seem difficult or intimidating—especially when it comes to certain subjects. Here are some tips to make it easier.

Talk About Everyday Stuff—And Do It Every Day

The more you do something, the easier it gets. Talking to the adults in your life about everyday stuff builds a bond that can smooth the way for when you need to discuss something more serious.

Find something trivial to chat about each day. Talk about how your team did at the track meet. Share something one of your teachers said. Even small talk about what's for dinner can keep your relationship strong and comfortable.

It's never too late to start. If you feel your relationship with your parents is strained, try easing into conversations. Mention that cute thing the dog did. Talk about how well your little sister is doing in math. Chatting with parents every day not only keeps an existing relationship strong, it also can help a frayed relationship get stronger.

About This Chapter: "Talking to Your Parents—or Other Adults," October 2012, reprinted with permission from www.kidshealth.org. This information was provided by KidsHealth®, one of the largest resources online for medically reviewed health information written for parents, kids, and teens. For more articles like this, visit www.KidsHealth.org or www.TeensHealth.org. Copyright © 1995–2012 The Nemours Foundation. All rights reserved.

When parents feel connected to your daily life, they can be there for you if something really important comes up.

Raising Difficult Topics

Maybe you need to break bad news to a parent, like getting a speeding ticket or failing an exam. Perhaps you're feeling scared or stressed about something. Or maybe you just really, really want to tell your parents about your new boyfriend or girlfriend, but you don't know how they'll react, how it will feel to tell them, or how to find the words.

Here are three steps to help you prepare for that talk.

Step 1: Know What You Want From The Conversation

It takes maturity to figure out what you want to get out of a conversation. (Most adults aren't so good at this!)

What you hope to achieve can vary. Most often you'll probably want the adults in your life to do one or more of these things:

- Simply listen and understand what you're going through without offering advice or commentary

- Give permission or support for something

- Offer you advice or help

- Guide you back on track if you're in trouble—in a way that's fair and without harsh criticism or put-downs

Why think about this before you begin talking? **So you can say why you want to talk in a way that communicates what you need.** For example:

- "Mom, I need to tell you about a problem I'm having, but I need you to just listen, OK? Don't give me advice—I just want you to know what's bothering me."

- "Dad, I need to get your permission to go on a class trip next week. Can I tell you about it?"

- "Grandad, I need your advice about something. Can we talk?"

Step 2: Identify Your Feelings

Things like personal feelings or sex are awkward to discuss with anyone, let alone a parent. It's natural to be nervous when talking about sensitive topics.

Recognize how you're feeling—for example, maybe you're worried that telling parents about a problem will make them disappointed or upset. **But instead of letting those feelings stop you from talking, put them into words as part of the conversation.** For example:

- "Mom, I need to talk to you—but I'm afraid I'll disappoint you."

- "Dad, I need to talk to you about something—but it's kind of embarrassing."

What if you think a parent may be unsupportive, harsh, or critical? It can help to defuse things by beginning with a statement like, "Mom, I have something to tell you. I'm not proud of what I've done, and you might be mad. But I know I need to tell you. Can you hear me out?"

Step 3: Pick A Good Time To Talk

Approach your parent when he or she isn't busy with something else. Ask, "Can we talk? Is now a good time?" Driving in the car or going for a walk can be great opportunities to talk. If it's hard to find a good time, say, "I need to talk to you. When is a good time?"

Difficult conversations benefit from good planning. **Think ahead about what you want to say or ask. Write down the most important ideas if you need to.**

How To Talk So Parents Will Listen

As most of us know, talking and listening don't go smoothly every time. Emotions and past experiences can get in the way.

Will parents take you seriously, believe what you say, listen to and respect your opinions, and hear you out without interrupting? A lot depends on your parent. Some parents are easy to talk to, some are great listeners, and some are harder to approach.

But some of what happens depends on you, too. **Since communication is a two-way street, the way you talk can influence how well a parent listens and understands you.**

So here are some guidelines to consider when talking to parents:

- **Be clear and direct.** Be as clear as you can about what you think, feel, and want. Give details that can help parents understand your situation. They can listen better or be more helpful if they understand what you mean and what's really going on.

- **Be honest.** If you're always honest, a parent will be likely to believe what you say. If you sometimes hide the truth or add too much drama, parents will have a harder time believing what you tell them. If you lie, they'll find it hard to trust you.

- **Try to understand their point of view.** If you have a disagreement, can you see your parents' side? If you can, say so. Telling parents you understand their views and feelings helps them be willing to see yours, too.

- **Try not to argue or whine.** Using a tone that's friendly and respectful makes it more likely parents will listen and take what you say seriously. It also makes it more likely that they'll talk to you in the same way. Of course, this is hard for any of us (adults included) when we're feeling heated about something. If you think your emotions might get the better of you, do something to blow off steam before talking: Go for a run. Cry. Hit your pillow. Do whatever it takes to sound calm when you need to.

What If Talking To Parents Doesn't Work?

Your parents won't always see things your way and they won't always say yes to what you ask. They might listen respectfully, understand your point of view, and do everything you need except say yes. It can be hard to take no for an answer. **But gracefully accepting a no can help you get more yeses in the future.**

What if it's more than just saying no to something, though? What if you really need your parents to be there for you but they can't? Some parents have troubles of their own. Others just can't be available in the ways their kids need and deserve. Others have a hard time being flexible.

If you can't talk to your parent, seek out other adults you can trust. Find a relative, a teacher, or a counselor who will listen, understand, encourage, believe in you, and care. Then follow all the tips above to get the most from your conversation with that person.

Acting respectfully demonstrates maturity. Parents are more likely to think of their children as grown up (and, as a result, capable of making more important decisions) when they see them acting maturely. Give these tips a try and you'll come across that way—maybe even more mature than your parents!

Chapter 46

Going To A Therapist

Eric went to therapy a couple of years ago when his parents were getting divorced. Although he no longer goes, he feels the two months he spent in therapy helped him get through the tough times as his parents worked out their differences.

Melody began seeing her therapist a year ago when she was being bullied at school. She still goes every two weeks because she feels therapy is really helping to build her self-esteem.

Britt just joined a therapy group for eating disorders led by her school's psychologist, and her friend Dana said she'd go with her.

When our parents were in school, very few kids went to therapy. Now it's much more common and also more accepted. Lots of teens wonder if therapy could help them.

Some Reasons Teens Go To Therapists

When teens are going through a rough time, such as family troubles or problems in school, they might feel more supported if they talk to a therapist. They may be feeling sad, angry, or overwhelmed by what's been happening—and need help sorting out their feelings, finding solutions to their problems, or just feeling better. That's when therapy can help.

Just a few examples of situations in which therapy can help are when someone:

- Feels sad, depressed, worried, shy, or just stressed out

About This Chapter: "Going to a Therapist," September 2010, reprinted with permission from www.kidshealth .org. This information was provided by KidsHealth®, one of the largest resources online for medically reviewed health information written for parents, kids, and teens. For more articles like this, visit www.KidsHealth.org or www.TeensHealth.org. Copyright © 1995–2012 The Nemours Foundation. All rights reserved.

- Is dieting or overeating for too long or it becomes a problem (eating disorders)

- Cuts, burns, or self-injures

- Is dealing with an attention problem (ADHD) or a learning problem

- Is coping with a chronic illness (such as diabetes or asthma) or a new diagnosis of a serious problem such as HIV, cancer, or a sexually transmitted disease (STD)

- Is dealing with family changes such as separation and divorce, or family problems such as alcoholism or addiction

- Is trying to cope with a traumatic event, death of a loved one, or worry over world events

- Has a habit he or she would like to get rid of, such as nail biting, hair pulling, smoking, or spending too much money, or getting hooked on medications, drugs, or pills

- Wants to sort out problems like managing anger or coping with peer pressure

- Wants to build self-confidence or figure out ways to make more friends

In short, therapy offers people support when they are going through difficult times.

Deciding to seek help for something you're going through can be really hard. It may be your idea to go to therapy or it might not. Sometimes parents or teachers bring up the idea first because they notice that someone they care about is dealing with a difficult situation, is losing weight, or seems unusually sad, worried, angry, or upset. Some people in this situation might welcome the idea or even feel relieved. Others might feel criticized or embarrassed and unsure if they'll benefit from talking to someone.

Sometimes people are told by teachers, parents, or the courts that they have to go see a therapist because they have been behaving in ways that are unacceptable, illegal, self-destructive, or dangerous. When therapy is someone else's idea, a person may at first feel like resisting the whole idea. But learning a bit more about what therapy involves and what to expect can help make it seem OK.

What Is Therapy?

Therapy isn't just for mental health. You've probably heard people discussing other types of medical therapy, such as physical therapy or chemotherapy. But the word "therapy" is most often used to mean psychotherapy (sometimes called "talk therapy")—in other words, psychological help to deal with stress or problems.

Psychotherapy is a process that's a lot like learning. Through therapy, people learn about themselves. They discover ways to overcome difficulties, develop inner strengths or skills, or make changes in themselves or their situations. Often, it feels good just to have a person to vent to, and other times it's useful to learn different techniques to help deal with stress.

A psychotherapist (therapist, for short) is a person who has been professionally trained to help people deal with stress or other problems. Psychiatrists, psychologists, social workers, counselors, and school psychologists are the titles of some of the licensed professionals who work as therapists. The letters following a therapist's name (for example, MD, PhD, PsyD, EdD, MA, LCSW, LPC) refer to the particular education and degree that therapist has received.

Some therapists specialize in working with a certain age group or on a particular type of problem. Other therapists treat a mix of ages and issues. Some work in hospitals, clinics, or counseling centers. Others work in schools or in psychotherapy offices, often called a "private practice" or "group practice."

What Do Therapists Do?

Most types of therapy include talking and listening, building trust, and receiving support and guidance. Sometimes therapists may recommend books for people to read or work through. They may also suggest keeping a journal. Some people prefer to express themselves using art or drawing. Others feel more comfortable just talking.

When a person talks to a therapist about which situations might be difficult for them or what stresses them out, this helps the therapist assess what is going on. The therapist and client then usually work together to set therapy goals and figure out what will help the person feel better or get back on track.

It might take a few meetings with a therapist before people really feel like they can share personal stuff. It's natural to feel that way. Trust is an essential ingredient in therapy—after all, therapy involves being open and honest about sensitive topics like feelings, ideas, relationships, problems, disappointments, and hopes. A therapist understands that people sometimes take a while to feel comfortable sharing personal information.

Most of the time, a person meets with a therapist one on one, which is known as individual therapy. Sometimes, though, a therapist might work with a family (called family therapy) or a group of people who all are dealing with similar issues (called group therapy or a support group). Family therapy gives family members a chance to talk together with a therapist about problems that involve them all. Group therapy and support groups help people give and receive support and learn from each other and their therapist by discussing the issues they have in common.

What Happens During Therapy?

If you see a therapist, he or she will talk with you about your feelings, thoughts, relationships, and important values. At the beginning, therapy sessions are focused on discussing what you'd like to work on and setting goals. Some of the goals people in therapy may set include things like:

- Improving self-esteem and gaining confidence

- Figuring out how to make more friends

- Feeling less depressed or less anxious

- Improving grades at school

- Learning to manage anger and frustration

- Making healthier choices (for example, about relationships or eating) and ending self-defeating behaviors

During the first visit, your therapist will probably ask you to talk a bit about yourself. Depending on your age, the therapist will also likely meet with a parent or caregiver and ask you to review information regarding confidentiality.

The first meeting can last longer than the usual "therapy hour" and is often called an "intake interview." This helps the therapist understand you better, and gives you a chance to see if you feel comfortable with the therapist. The therapist will probably ask about problems, concerns, and symptoms that you may be having, or the problems that parents or teachers are concerned about.

After one or two sessions, the therapist may talk to you about his or her understanding of what is going on with you, how therapy could help, and what the process will involve. Together, you and your therapist will decide on the goals for therapy and how frequently to meet. This may be once a week, every other week, or once a month.

With a better understanding of your situation, the therapist might teach you new skills or help you to think about a situation in a new way. For example, therapists can help people develop better relationship skills or coping skills, including ways to build confidence, express feelings, or manage anger.

Sticking to the schedule you agree on with your therapist and going to your appointments will ensure you have enough time with your therapist to work out your concerns. If your therapist suggests a schedule that you don't think you'll be able to keep, be up front about it so you can work out an alternative.

Can I get over depression without taking medication?

I've been depressed for a while. It has affected my schoolwork and social life a lot. How can I get over being depressed without taking antidepressants? —Sara*

Not everyone who's depressed needs to take antidepressant medications. There are many other things that can help. Finding out what's best for you starts with an evaluation by your doctor or qualified therapist.

Talk therapy (a very common treatment for depression) helps people give words to sad feelings, talk about their situation, and feel understood. Therapy also helps people learn how to turn thoughts in a more positive direction and come up with ways to work out problems.

Don't underestimate the power of seemingly simple actions to help put your mood back in balance. Get outside. Take a walk. Play a sport you enjoy. Choose nutritious foods and resist junk foods. Get a full night's sleep. People who are depressed may not feel much like being active. But make yourself do it anyway (ask a friend to exercise with you if you need to be motivated).

For people who experience seasonal wintertime depression, getting enough daylight is important. This can be done by getting outdoors every day or by using a special type of light box.

It's common for depression to have an impact on social life because it can make a person feel withdrawn and subdued. Try to spend time with a good friend doing something you both enjoy or just hanging out. Open up to someone you feel close to—a friend or parent. Let someone know what's going on with you. Don't dwell on troubles—share the good parts of your day, too. It's the sharing that matters. Feeling connected to others helps relieve depression.

Above all, be kind to yourself. Depression affects a person's thoughts, making everything seem dismal, negative, and hopeless. Don't let this translate into down-on-yourself thinking. Try to remember your strengths, gifts, and blessings.

Some people do need medication to get over depression. But it is rarely used alone as a treatment—especially in young people. How will you know what is best for you? See your doctor or therapist for an evaluation and a treatment plan that's right for you.

*Names have been changed to protect user privacy.

How Private Is It?

Therapists respect the privacy of their clients and they keep things they're told confidential. A therapist won't tell anyone else—including parents—about what a person discusses in his or her sessions unless that person gives permission. The only exception is if therapists believe their clients may harm themselves or others.

If the issue of privacy and confidentiality worries you, be sure to ask your therapist about it during your first meeting. It's important to feel comfortable with your therapist so you can talk openly about your situation.

Does It Mean I'm Crazy?

No. In fact, many people in your class have probably seen a therapist at some point—just like students often see tutors or coaches for extra help with schoolwork or sports. Getting help in dealing with emotions and stressful situations is as important to your overall health as getting help with a medical problem like asthma or diabetes.

There's nothing wrong with getting help with problems that are hard to solve alone. In fact, it's just the opposite. It takes a lot of courage and maturity to look for solutions to problems instead of ignoring or hiding them and allowing them to become worse. If you think that therapy could help you with a problem, ask an adult you trust—like a parent, school counselor, or doctor—to help you find a therapist.

A few adults still resist the idea of therapy because they don't fully understand it or have outdated ideas about it. A couple of generations ago, people didn't know as much about the mind or the mind-body connection as they do today, and people were left to struggle with their problems on their own. It used to be that therapy was only available to those with the most serious mental health problems, but that's no longer the case.

Therapy is helpful to people of all ages and with problems that range from mild to much more serious. Some people still hold on to old beliefs about therapy, such as thinking that teens "will grow out of" their problems. If the adults in your family don't seem open to talking about therapy, mention your concerns to a school counselor, coach, or doctor.

You don't have to hide the fact that you're going to a therapist, but you also don't have to tell anyone if you'd prefer not to. Some people find that talking to a few close friends about their therapy helps them to work out their problems and feel like they're not alone. Other people choose not to tell anyone, especially if they feel that others won't understand. Either way, it's a personal decision.

What Can A Person Get Out Of Therapy?

What someone gets out of therapy depends on why that person is there. For example, some people go to therapy to solve a specific problem, others want to begin making better choices, and others want to start to heal from a loss or a difficult life situation.

Therapy can help people feel better, be stronger, and make good choices as well as discover more about themselves. Those who work with therapists might learn about motivations that lead them to behave in certain ways or about inner strengths they have. Maybe you'll learn new coping skills, develop more patience, or learn to like yourself better. Maybe you'll find new ways to handle problems that come up or new ways to handle yourself in tough situations.

People who work with therapists often find that they learn a lot about themselves and that therapy can help them grow and mature. Lots of people discover that the tools they learn in therapy when they're young make them feel stronger and better able to deal with whatever life throws at them even as adults. If you are curious about the therapy process, talk to a counselor or therapist to see if you could benefit.

Chapter 47

Handle Your Anger

Do you have a short fuse or find yourself getting into frequent arguments and fights? Anger is a normal, healthy emotion, but when chronic, explosive anger spirals out of control, it can have serious consequences for your relationships, your health, and your state of mind. With insight about the real reasons for your anger and these anger management tools, you can learn to keep your temper from hijacking your life.

Understanding Anger

The emotion of anger is neither good nor bad. It's perfectly healthy and normal to feel angry when you've been mistreated or wronged. The feeling isn't the problem—it's what you do with it that makes a difference. Anger becomes a problem when it harms you or others.

If you have a hot temper, you may feel like it's out of your hands and there's little you can do to tame the beast. But you have more control over your anger than you think. You can learn to express your emotions without hurting others—and when you do, you'll not only feel better, you'll also be more likely to get your needs met. Mastering the art of anger management takes work, but the more you practice, the easier it will get. And the payoff can be huge. Learning to control your anger and express it appropriately can help you build better relationships, achieve your goals, and lead a healthier, more satisfying life.

About This Chapter: "Anger Management: Tips and Techniques for Getting Anger Under Control," by Jeanne Segal, Ph.D. and Melinda Smith, M.A., updated March 2013. © 2013 Helpguide.org. All rights reserved. Helpguide provides a detailed list of references and resources for this article, with links to related Helpguide topics and information from other websites. For a complete list of these resources, go to http://www.helpguide .org/mental/anger_management_control_tips_techniques.htm.

Myths And Facts About Anger

Myth: I shouldn't "hold in" my anger. It's healthy to vent and let it out.

Fact: While it's true that suppressing and ignoring anger is unhealthy, venting is no better. Anger is not something you have to "let out" in an aggressive way in order to avoid blowing up. In fact, outbursts and tirades only fuel the fire and reinforce your anger problem.

Myth: Anger, aggression, and intimidation help me earn respect and get what I want.

Fact: True power doesn't come from bullying others. People may be afraid of you, but they won't respect you if you can't control yourself or handle opposing viewpoints. Others will be more willing to listen to you and accommodate your needs if you communicate in a respectful way.

Myth: I can't help myself. Anger isn't something you can control.

Fact: You can't always control the situation you're in or how it makes you feel, but you can control how you express your anger. And you can express your anger without being verbally or physically abusive. Even if someone is pushing your buttons, you always have a choice about how to respond.

Myth: Anger management is about learning to suppress your anger.

Fact: Never getting angry is not a good goal. Anger is normal, and it will come out regardless of how hard you try to suppress it. Anger management is all about becoming aware of your underlying feelings and needs and developing healthier ways to manage upset. Rather than trying to suppress your anger, the goal is to express it in constructive ways.

Source: "Anger Management: Tips and Techniques for Getting Anger Under Control." © 2013 Helpguide.org. All rights reserved.

Why Learning To Control Your Anger Is Important

You might think that venting your anger is healthy, that the people around you are too sensitive, that your anger is justified, or that you need to show your fury to get respect. But the truth is that anger is much more likely to damage your relationships, impair your judgment, get in the way of success, and have a negative impact on the way people see you.

- **Out-of-control anger hurts your physical health**. Constantly operating at high levels of stress and tension is bad for your health. Chronic anger makes you more susceptible to heart disease, diabetes, high cholesterol levels, a weakened immune system, insomnia, and high blood pressure.

- **Out-of-control anger hurts your mental health.** Chronic anger consumes huge amounts of mental energy and clouds your thinking, making it harder to concentrate, see the bigger picture, and enjoy life. It can also lead to stress, depression, and other mental health problems.

- **Out-of-control anger hurts your career.** Constructive criticism, creative differences, and heated debate can be healthy. But lashing out only alienates your colleagues, supervisors, or clients and erodes their respect. What's more, a bad reputation can follow you wherever you go, making it harder and harder to get ahead.

- **Out-of-control anger hurts your relationships with others.** It causes lasting scars in the people you love most and gets in the way of your friendships and work relationships. Chronic, intense anger makes it hard for others to trust you, speak honestly, or feel comfortable—they never know what is going to set you off or what you will do. Explosive anger is especially damaging to children.

Anger Control And Management Tip 1: Explore What's Really Behind Your Anger

If you're struggling with out-of-control anger, you may be wondering why your fuse is so short. Anger problems often stem from what you've learned as a child.

If you watched others in your family scream, hit each other, or throw things, you might think this is how anger is supposed to be expressed. Traumatic events and high levels of stress can make you more susceptible to anger as well.

Anger Is Often A Cover-Up For Other Feelings

In order to get your needs met and express your anger in appropriate ways, you need to be in touch with what you are really feeling. Are you truly angry? Or is your anger masking other feelings such as embarrassment, insecurity, hurt, shame, or vulnerability?

If your knee-jerk response in many situations is anger, it is very likely that your temper is covering up your true feelings and needs. This is especially likely if you grew up in a family where expressing feelings was strongly discouraged. As an adult, you may have a hard time acknowledging feelings other than anger.

Clues That There's Something More To Your Anger

- **You have a hard time compromising.** Is it hard for you to understand other people's points of view, and even harder to concede a point? If you grew up in a family where anger was out of control, you may remember how the angry person got his or her way by being the loudest and most demanding. Compromising might bring up scary feelings of failure and vulnerability.

- **You have trouble expressing emotions other than anger.** Do you pride yourself on being tough and in control, never letting your guard down? Do you feel that emotions like fear, guilt, or shame don't apply to you? Everyone has those emotions, and if you think you don't, you may be using anger as a cover for them.

- **You view different opinions and viewpoints as a personal challenge to you.** Do you believe that your way is always right and get angry when others disagree? If you have a strong need to be in control or a fragile ego, you may interpret other perspectives as a challenge to your authority, rather than simply a different way of looking at things.

If you are uncomfortable with many emotions, disconnected, or stuck on an angry one-note response to everything, it might do you some good to get back in touch with your feelings.

Emotional awareness is the key to self-understanding and success in life. Without the ability to recognize, manage, and deal with the full range of human emotions, you'll inevitably spin into confusion, isolation, and self-doubt.

Some Dynamics Of Anger

- We become more angry when we are stressed and body resources are down.
- We are rarely ever angry for the reasons we think.
- We are often angry when we didn't get what we needed as a child.
- We often become angry when we see a trait in others we can't stand in ourselves.
- Underneath many current angers are old disappointments, traumas, and triggers.
- Sometimes we get angry because we were hurt as a child.
- We get angry when a current event brings up an old unresolved situation from the past.
- We often feel strong emotion when a situation has a similar content, words or energy that we have felt before.

Anger Control And Management Tip 2: Be Aware Of Your Anger Warning Signs And Triggers

While you might feel that you just explode into anger without warning, in fact, there are physical warning signs in your body. Anger is a normal physical response. It fuels the "fight or flight" system of the body, and the angrier you get, the more your body goes into overdrive. Becoming aware of your own personal signs that your temper is starting to boil allows you to take steps to manage your anger before it gets out of control.

Pay Attention To The Way Anger Feels In Your Body

- Knots in your stomach
- Clenching your hands or jaw
- Feeling clammy or flushed
- Breathing faster
- Headaches
- Pacing or needing to walk around
- "Seeing red"
- Having trouble concentrating
- Pounding heart
- Tensing your shoulders

Identify The Negative Thought Patterns That Trigger Your Temper

You may think that external things—the insensitive actions of other people, for example, or frustrating situations—are what cause your anger. But anger problems have less to do with what happens to you than how you interpret and think about what happened. Common negative thinking patterns that trigger and fuel anger include:

- **Overgeneralizing:** For example, "You always interrupt me. You NEVER consider my needs. EVERYONE disrespects me. I NEVER get the credit I deserve."

- **Obsessing on "shoulds" and "musts:"** Having a rigid view of the way things should or must be and getting angry when reality doesn't line up with this vision.

- **Mind reading and jumping to conclusions:** Assuming you "know" what someone else is thinking or feeling—that he or she intentionally upset you, ignored your wishes, or disrespected you.

- **Collecting straws:** Looking for things to get upset about, usually while overlooking or blowing past anything positive. Letting these small irritations build and build until you reach the "final straw" and explode, often over something relatively minor.

- **Blaming:** When anything bad happens or something goes wrong, it's always someone else's fault. You blame others for the things that happen to you rather than taking responsibility for your own life.

Avoid People, Places, And Situations That Bring Out Your Worst

Stressful events don't excuse anger, but understanding how these events affect you can help you take control of your environment and avoid unnecessary aggravation. Look at your regular routine and try to identify activities, times of day, people, places, or situations that trigger irritable or angry feelings. Maybe you get into a fight every time you go out for drinks with a certain group of friends.

Or maybe the traffic on your daily commute drives you crazy. Then, think about ways to avoid these triggers or view the situation differently so it doesn't make your blood boil.

Anger Control And Management Tip 3: Learn Ways To Cool Down

Once you know how to recognize the warning signs that your temper is rising and anticipate your triggers, you can act quickly to deal with your anger before it spins out of control. There are many techniques that can help you cool down and keep your anger in check.

Quick Tips For Cooling Down

- **Focus on the physical sensations of anger.** While it may seem counterintuitive, tuning into the way your body feels when you're angry often lessens the emotional intensity of your anger.

- **Take some deep breaths.** Deep, slow breathing helps counteract rising tension. The key is to breathe deeply from the abdomen, getting as much fresh air as possible into your lungs.

- **Exercise.** A brisk walk around the block is a great idea. It releases pent-up energy so you can approach the situation with a cooler head.

- **Use your senses.** Take advantage of the relaxing power of your sense of sight, smell, hearing, touch, and taste. You might try listening to music or picturing yourself in a favorite place.

- **Stretch or massage areas of tension.** Roll your shoulders if you are tensing them, for example, or gently massage your neck and scalp.

- **Slowly count to ten.** Focus on the counting to let your rational mind catch up with your feelings. If you still feel out of control by the time you reach ten, start counting again.

Give Yourself A Reality Check

When you start getting upset about something, take a moment to think about the situation. Ask yourself:

- How important is it in the grand scheme of things?

- Is it really worth getting angry about it?

- Is it worth ruining the rest of my day?

- Is my response appropriate to the situation?

- Is there anything I can do about it?

- Is taking action worth my time?

Anger Control And Management Tip 4: Find Healthier Ways To Express Your Anger

If you've decided that the situation is worth getting angry about and there's something you can do to make it better, the key is to express your feelings in a healthy way. When communicated respectfully and channeled effectively, anger can be a tremendous source of energy and inspiration for change.

Pinpoint What You're Really Angry About

Have you ever gotten into an argument over something silly? Big fights often happen over something small, like a dish left out or being ten minutes late. But there's usually a bigger issue behind it. If you find your irritation and anger rapidly rising, ask yourself, "What am I really angry about?" Identifying the real source of frustration will help you communicate your anger better, take constructive action, and work towards a resolution.

Take Five If Things Get Too Heated

If your anger seems to be spiraling out of control, remove yourself from the situation for a few minutes or for as long as it takes you to cool down. A brisk walk, a trip to the gym, or a few minutes listening to some music should allow you to calm down, release pent up emotion, and then approach the situation with a cooler head.

Always Fight Fair

It's okay to be upset at someone, but if you don't fight fair, the relationship will quickly breakdown. Fighting fair allows you to express your own needs while still respecting others.

What can I do if I want to be more assertive?

Being assertive means that you respect yourself and others equally and that you portray this in the way you communicate and respond to other people. Being assertive means that you are able to "stand up" for yourself and others. When you are assertive, you are better able to stand up to a bully and you are better able to say no to peer pressure.

There are three response styles:

- Passive
- Aggressive
- Assertive

A passive response is to behave as if other people's rights and opinions are more important than your own.

An aggressive response is to behave as if your rights and opinions are more important than those of other people.

An assertive response is to respect yourself and others equally.

The thoughts we each have about ourselves can help or hinder us. Sometimes we may put ourselves down saying "no one will like me," "I am hopeless at this," etc. We can change this and instead say helpful things about ourselves, like "I have the right to ask for what I want," "I did OK," or "It wasn't perfect, but it was OK."

Sometimes we may describe ourselves as "timid," "shy," "pushy," or "bossy." By being assertive, we can let others know what we want and how we feel, without being pushy or bossy, and still not be too shy or afraid to speak up.

Being assertive is always important. It is especially important if:

1. You are being bullied;
2. Your friend is being bullied; [and/or]
3. You are being pressured to do something you don't want to do.

- **Make the relationship your priority.** Maintaining and strengthening the relationship, rather than "winning" the argument, should always be your first priority. Be respectful of the other person and his or her viewpoint.

- **Focus on the present.** Once you are in the heat of arguing, it's easy to start throwing past grievances into the mix. Rather than looking to the past and assigning blame, focus on what you can do in the present to solve the problem.

How To Be Assertive

1. Use "I" messages: "I" messages let you say what you think and how you feel without putting down or attacking the other person. When you are hurt, upset, or angry, an "I" message can help. An "I" message has three basic parts:

- **I feel:** Tell how you feel. Follow "I feel" with a feeling word, [such as] "**I feel** disappointed."
- **When:** Tell what the other person did or said that caused you to feel that way. "I feel disappointed **when** you cancel our plans at the last minute."
- **I want:** Tell what you want to happen: "I feel disappointed when you cancel our plans at the last minute. **I want** you to let me know earlier if you can't make it."

An "I" message can include a fourth part telling why you feel as you do about what happened.

- **Because:** [Tell why you feel as you do.] "I feel disappointed when you cancel our plans at the last minute, **because** then I'm left on my own and it's too late to plan something else. I want you to let me know earlier if you can't make it."

2. Be clear about what you want. Know what you want to say and practice it. Make your request short: "That is mine. I want you to give it back."

3. Be a broken record. A broken record repeats the same thing over and over. Know what you want to say and stick to it: "That is my pencil and I want it back." It is possible to respond kindly first before repeating the statement: "I am sorry you have no pencil, but that is my pencil and I want it back." (A possible broken record response to being teased: "I am sorry, I didn't hear you.")

4. Say no. If you are not sure if you want to do something, you can say: "I don't know. I need more time or more information." If you know your answer is no, then say "No." Try not to be indecisive. Try not to be persuaded to do what you don't want to do. You can offer an alternative: "No, I don't want to go to the party. Let's go to a movie instead."

5. Keep good eye contact. Practice walking tall in front of a mirror. Practice keeping eye contact with people.

Source: "What Can I Do to Be More Assertive?" reprinted with permission from the Department of Education, Government of Newfoundland and Labrador, http://www.ed.gov.nl.ca. Copyright Government of Newfoundland and Labrador, 2013. All rights reserved.

- **Choose your battles.** Conflicts can be draining, so it's important to consider whether the issue is really worthy of your time and energy. If you pick your battles rather than fighting over every little thing, others will take you more seriously when you are upset.

- **Be willing to forgive.** Resolving conflict is impossible if you're unwilling or unable to forgive. Resolution lies in releasing the urge to punish, which can never compensate for our losses and only adds to our injury by further depleting and draining our lives.

- **Know when to let something go.** If you can't come to an agreement, agree to disagree. It takes two people to keep an argument going. If a conflict is going nowhere, you can choose to disengage and move on.

Developing Your Conflict Resolution Skills

The way you respond to differences and disagreements at home and at work can create hostility and irreparable rifts, or it can build safety and trust. Learning how to resolve conflict in a positive way will help you strengthen your relationships.

When To Seek Help For Anger Management

If your anger is still spiraling out of control, despite putting the previous anger management techniques into practice, or if you're getting into trouble with the law or hurting others—you need more help. There are many therapists, classes, and programs for people with anger management problems. Asking for help is not a sign of weakness. You'll often find others in the same shoes, and getting direct feedback on techniques for controlling anger can be tremendously helpful.

- **Therapy for anger problems:** Therapy can be a great way to explore the reasons behind your anger. If you don't know why you are getting angry, it's very hard to control. Therapy provides a safe environment to learn more about your reasons and identify triggers for your anger. It's also a safe place to practice new skills in expressing your anger.

- **Anger management classes or groups:** Anger management classes or groups allow you to see others coping with the same struggles. You will also learn tips and techniques for managing your anger and hear other people's stories. For domestic violence issues, traditional anger management is usually not recommended. There are special classes that go to the issue of power and control that are at the heart of domestic violence.

If Your Loved One Has An Anger Management Problem

If your loved one has an anger problem, you probably feel like you're walking on eggshells all the time. But always remember that you are not to blame for your loved one's anger. There is never an excuse for physically or verbally abusive behavior. You have a right to be treated with respect and to live without fear of an angry outburst or a violent rage.

Tips For Dealing With A Loved One's Anger Management Problem

While you can't control another person's anger, you can control how you respond to it:

- Set clear boundaries about what you will and will not tolerate.
- Wait for a time when you are both calm to talk to your loved one about the anger problem.
- Don't bring it up when either one of you is already angry.
- Remove yourself from the situation if your loved one does not calm down.
- Consider counseling or therapy for yourself if you are having a hard time standing up for yourself.
- Put your safety first. Trust your instincts. If you feel unsafe or threatened in any way, get away from your loved one and go somewhere safe.

Anger Isn't The Real Problem In Abusive Relationships

Despite what many people believe, domestic violence and abuse is not due to the abuser's loss of control over his behavior and temper. In fact, abusive behavior is a deliberate choice for

Consider Professional Help If:

- You feel constantly frustrated and angry no matter what you try.
- Your temper causes problems at work or in your relationships.
- You avoid new events and people because you feel like you can't control your temper.
- You have gotten in trouble with the law due to your anger.
- Your anger has ever led to physical violence.

Source: Source: "Anger Management: Tips and Techniques for Getting Anger Under Control." © 2013 Helpguide.org. All rights reserved.

the sole purpose of controlling you. If you are in an abusive relationship, know that couples counseling is not recommended—and that your partner needs specialized treatment, not regular anger management classes.

Chapter 48

Body Image And Self-Esteem

Does any of this sound familiar? "I'm too tall." "I'm too short." "I'm too skinny." "If only I was shorter/taller/had curly hair/straight hair/a smaller nose/longer legs, I'd be happy."

Are you putting yourself down? If so, you're not alone. As a teen, you're going through lots of changes in your body. And, as your body changes, so does your image of yourself. It's not always easy to like every part of your looks, but when you get stuck on the negatives it can really bring down your self-esteem.

Why Are Self-Esteem And Body Image Important?

Self-esteem is all about how much you feel you are worth—and how much you feel other people value you. Self-esteem is important because feeling good about yourself can affect your mental health and how you behave.

People with high self-esteem know themselves well. They're realistic and find friends that like and appreciate them for who they are. People with high self-esteem usually feel more in control of their lives and know their own strengths and weaknesses.

Body image is how you view your physical self—including whether you feel you are attractive and whether others like your looks. For many people, especially people in their early teens, body image can be closely linked to self-esteem.

What Influences A Person's Self-Esteem?

Puberty And Development

Some people struggle with their self-esteem and body image when they begin puberty because it's a time when the body goes through many changes. These changes, combined with wanting to feel accepted by our friends, means it can be tempting to compare ourselves with others. The trouble with that is, not everyone grows or develops at the same time or in the same way.

Media Images And Other Outside Influences

Our tweens and early teens are a time when we become more aware of celebrities and media images—as well as how other kids look and how we fit in. We might start to compare ourselves with other people or media images ("ideals" that are frequently airbrushed). All of this can affect how we feel about ourselves and our bodies even as we grow into our teens.

Families And School

Family life can sometimes influence our body image. Some parents or coaches might be too focused on looking a certain way or "making weight" for a sports team. Family members might struggle with their own body image or criticize their kids' looks ("why do you wear your hair so long?" or "how come you can't wear pants that fit you?"). This can all influence a person's self-esteem, especially if they're sensitive to others peoples' comments.

People also may experience negative comments and hurtful teasing about the way they look from classmates and peers. Although these often come from ignorance, sometimes they can affect body image and self-esteem.

Healthy Self-Esteem

If you have a positive body image, you probably like and accept yourself the way you are, even if you don't fit some media "ideal." This healthy attitude allows you to explore other aspects of growing up, such as developing good friendships, becoming more independent from your parents, and challenging yourself physically and mentally. Developing these parts of yourself can help boost your self-esteem.

A positive, optimistic attitude can help people develop strong self-esteem. For example, if you make a mistake, you might want to say, "Hey, I'm human" instead of "Wow, I'm such a loser" or not blame others when things don't go as expected.

> ## Resilience
>
> People who believe in themselves are better able to recognize mistakes, learn from them, and bounce back from disappointment. This skill is called resilience.

Knowing what makes you happy and how to meet your goals can help you feel capable, strong, and in control of your life. A positive attitude and a healthy lifestyle (such as exercising and eating right) are a great combination for building good self-esteem.

Tips For Improving Body Image

Some people think they need to change how they look to feel good about themselves. But all you need to do is change the way you see your body and how you think about yourself. Here are some tips on doing that:

Recognize that your body is your own, no matter what shape or size it comes in. Try to focus on how strong and healthy your body is and the things it can do, not what's wrong with it or what you feel you want to change about it. If you're worried about your weight or size, check with your doctor to verify that things are OK. But it's no one's business but your own what your body is like—ultimately, you have to be happy with yourself.

Identify which aspects of your appearance you can realistically change and which you can't. Humans, by definition, are imperfect. It's what makes each of us unique and original! Everyone (even the most perfect-seeming celeb) has things that they can't change and need to accept—like their height, for example, or their shoe size. Remind yourself that "real people aren't perfect and perfect people aren't real (they're usually airbrushed!)".

If there are things about yourself that you want to change and can, do this by making goals for yourself. For example, if you want to get fit, make a plan to exercise every day and eat healthy. Then keep track of your progress until you reach your goal. Meeting a challenge you set for yourself is a great way to boost self-esteem!

When you hear negative comments coming from within, tell yourself to stop. Appreciate that each person is more than just how he or she looks on any given day. We're complex and constantly changing. Try to focus on what's unique and interesting about yourself.

Try building your self-esteem by giving yourself three compliments every day. While you're at it, every evening list three things in your day that really gave you pleasure. It can be anything from the way the sun felt on your face, the sound of your favorite band, or the way someone laughed at your jokes. By focusing on the good things you do and the positive aspects of your life, you can change how you feel about yourself.

Some people with physical disabilities or differences may feel they are not seen for their true selves because of their bodies and what they can and can't do. Other people may have such serious body image issues that they need a bit more help. Working with a counselor or therapist can help some people gain perspective and learn to focus on their individual strengths as well as develop healthier thinking.

Where Can I Go If I Need Help?

Sometimes low self-esteem and body image problems are too much to handle alone. A few teens may become depressed, and lose interest in activities or friends. Some go on to develop eating or body image disorders, and can become depressed or use alcohol or drugs to escape feelings of low worth.

If you're feeling this way, it can help to talk to a parent, coach, religious leader, guidance counselor, therapist, or friend. A trusted adult—someone who supports you and doesn't bring you down—can help you put your body image in perspective and give you positive feedback about your body, your skills, and your abilities.

If you can't turn to anyone you know, call a teen crisis hotline (an online search can give you the information for national and local hotlines). The most important thing is to get help if you feel like your body image and self-esteem are affecting your life.

Chapter 49

Exercise Is Wise

You've probably heard countless times how exercise is "good for you." But did you know that it can actually help you feel good, too? Getting the right amount of exercise can rev up your energy levels and even help improve your mood.

Rewards And Benefits

Experts recommend that teens get 60 minutes or more of moderate to vigorous physical activity each day. Here are some of the reasons:

- **Exercise benefits every part of the body, including the mind.** Exercising causes the body to produce endorphins, chemicals that can help a person to feel more peaceful and happy. Exercise can help some people sleep better. It can also help some people who have mild depression and low self-esteem. Plus, exercise can give people a real sense of accomplishment and pride at having achieved a certain goal—like beating an old time in the 100-meter dash.

- **Exercising can help you look better.** People who exercise burn more calories and look more toned than those who don't. In fact, exercise is one of the most important parts of keeping your body at a healthy weight.

- **Exercise helps people lose weight and lower the risk of some diseases.** Exercising to maintain a healthy weight decreases a person's risk of developing certain diseases,

About This Chapter: "Why Exercise Is Wise," July 2012, reprinted with permission fromwww.kidshealth.org. This information was provided by KidsHealth®, one of the largest resources online for medically reviewed health information written for parents, kids, and teens. For more articles like this, visitwww.KidsHealth.org or www .TeensHealth.org.Copyright © 1995–2012 The Nemours Foundation. All rights reserved.

including type 2 diabetes and high blood pressure. These diseases, which used to be found mostly in adults, are becoming more common in teens.

- **Exercise can help a person age well.** This may not seem important now, but your body will thank you later. Women are especially prone to a condition called osteoporosis (a weakening of the bones) as they get older. Studies have found that weight-bearing exercise—like jumping, running, or brisk walking—can help girls (and guys!) keep their bones strong.

The three components to a well-balanced exercise routine are: aerobic exercise, strength training, and flexibility training.

Aerobic Exercise

Like other muscles, the heart enjoys a good workout. You can provide it with one in the form of aerobic exercise. Aerobic exercise is any type of exercise that gets the heart pumping and quickens your breathing. When you give your heart this kind of workout regularly, it will get stronger and more efficient in delivering oxygen (in the form of oxygen-carrying blood cells) to all parts of your body.

If you play team sports, you're probably meeting the recommendation for 60 minutes or more of moderate to vigorous activity on practice days. Some team sports that give you a great aerobic workout are swimming, basketball, soccer, lacrosse, hockey, and rowing.

But if you don't play team sports, don't worry—there are plenty of ways to get aerobic exercise on your own or with friends. These include biking, running, swimming, dancing, in-line skating, tennis, cross-country skiing, hiking, and walking quickly. In fact, the types of exercise that you do on your own are easier to continue when you leave high school and go on to work or college, making it easier to stay fit later in life as well.

Strength Training

The heart isn't the only muscle to benefit from regular exercise. Most of the other muscles in your body enjoy exercise, too. When you use your muscles and they become stronger, it allows you to be active for longer periods of time without getting worn out.

Strong muscles are also a plus because they actually help protect you when you exercise by supporting your joints and helping to prevent injuries. Muscle also burns more energy when a person's at rest than fat does, so building your muscles will help you burn more calories and maintain a healthy weight.

Different types of exercise strengthen different muscle groups, for example:

- For arms, try rowing or cross-country skiing. Pull-ups and push-ups, those old gym class standbys, are also good for building arm muscles.

- For strong legs, try running, biking, rowing, or skating. Squats and leg raises also work the legs.

- For shapely abs, you can't beat rowing, yoga or Pilates, and crunches.

Flexibility Training

Strengthening the heart and other muscles isn't the only important goal of exercise. Exercise also helps the body stay flexible, meaning that your muscles and joints stretch and bend easily. People who are flexible can worry less about strained muscles and sprains.

Being flexible may also help improve a person's sports performance. Some activities, like dance or martial arts, obviously require great flexibility, but increased flexibility can also help people perform better at other sports, such as soccer or lacrosse.

Sports and activities that encourage flexibility are easy to find. Martial arts like karate also help a person stay flexible. Ballet, gymnastics, Pilates, and yoga are other good choices. Stretching after your workout will also help you improve your flexibility.

What's Right For Me?

One of the biggest reasons people drop an exercise program is lack of interest: If what you're doing isn't fun, it's hard to keep it up. The good news is that there are tons of different sports and activities that you can try out to see which one inspires you.

When picking the right type of exercise, it can help to consider your workout personality. For example, do you like to work out alone and on your own schedule? If so, solo sports like biking or snowboarding may be for you. Or do you like the shared motivation and companionship that comes from being part of a team?

You also need to plan around practical considerations, such as whether your chosen activity is affordable and available to you. (Activities like horseback riding may be harder for people who live in cities, for example.) You'll also want to think about how much time you can set aside for your sport.

It's a good idea to talk to someone who understands the exercise, like a coach or fitness expert at a gym. He or she can get you started on a program that's right for you and your level of fitness.

Another thing to consider is whether any health conditions may affect how—and how much—you exercise. Doctors know that most people benefit from regular exercise, even those with disabilities or conditions like asthma. But if you have a health problem or other considerations (like being overweight or very out of shape), talk to your doctor before beginning an exercise plan. That way you can get information on which exercise programs are best and which to avoid.

Why Fitness Matters

Exercise is an important part of a lifetime of good health! Exercising is also fun and is something you can do with friends. Regular exercise provides both mental and physical health benefits.

Mental Health Benefits Of Exercise

One of the great things about exercise is that it can improve your mental health. Regular exercise can help you feel less stressed, can improve your self-esteem, and can help you to feel ready to learn in school. Kids who exercise may also have reduced symptoms of anxiety and depression.

Exercise can also improve your overall mood. Did you have an argument with a friend? Or did you do poorly on a test? A workout at the gym or a brisk 30-minute walk will make your brain produce chemicals that will make you happier and more relaxed than before you started working out.

What if you're having trouble sleeping? Again, it's exercise to the rescue! Regular exercise can help you fall asleep faster and help you sleep deeper. A good night's sleep can improve your concentration and productivity in school the next day.

Physical Health Benefits Of Exercise

Another great thing about exercise is that it can keep your body healthy. Kids who exercise often have a healthier body weight than kids who don't exercise. Exercise makes your bones solid, improves your heart and lungs, and makes your muscles strong.

Exercise can also affect specific diseases that affect adolescents and teens. New research shows that teens who exercise regularly (about 60 minutes of brisk exercise each day) burn more calories and use blood sugar more efficiently than teens who don't exercise. This could protect you from developing type 2 diabetes. Why should this concern you? Well, in recent years, a lot of health problems that doctors saw only in adults are now seen in young people. For example,

Too Much Of A Good Thing

As with all good things, it's possible to overdo exercise. Although exercising is a great way to maintain a healthy weight, exercising too much to lose weight isn't healthy. The body needs enough calories to function properly. This is especially true for teens, who are still growing.

15 years ago type 2 diabetes was rare among adolescents, but now it accounts for almost 50 percent of new cases of diabetes in young people. In fact, type 2 diabetes used to be called "adult-onset diabetes," but the name was changed because so many young people were developing the disease.

Here is something else to consider: Children and adolescents who are overweight are more likely to become adults who are overweight. If you start good habits (like daily exercise) when you are young, you will be likely to continue them when you're older.

New research shows that exercise during the teen years (beginning at age 12) can help protect girls from breast cancer when they are older. Also, regular physical activity can help prevent colon cancer later in your life.

Get Moving!

The more time you spend in front of the television or playing video games, the less time you have to be active. Not being active is called sedentary (say: sed-un-tair-ee). Leading a sedentary lifestyle can cause weight gain and even obesity (dangerously high weight), which can lead to type 2 diabetes, high cholesterol levels, and high blood pressure. These three health issues can hurt your heart and make it easier for you to get certain diseases. Make physical activity a regular part of your life. It can help you protect your health! Obesity can also hurt your self-esteem, too.

What is physical fitness? A condition or state of being that helps you look, feel, and do your best. It is the ability to do tasks full of energy, and still be able to do other things with your time, such as schoolwork and activities with family and friends. It is a basis for good health and well-being. Fitness involves performance of the heart and lungs, and the muscles of the body. Fitness can also influence how alert you are and how you feel emotionally.

Source: "Fitness: Why Fitness Matters," U.S. Department of Health and Human Services, Office on Women's Health (www.girlshealth.gov), October 2009.

307

Exercising too much in an effort to burn calories and lose weight (also called compulsive exercise) can be a sign of an eating disorder. If you ever get the feeling that your exercise is in charge of you rather than the other way around, talk with your doctor, a parent, or another adult you trust.

It's also possible to over train—something high school athletes need to watch out for. If you participate in one sport, experts recommend that you limit that activity to a maximum of five days a week, with at least 2–3 months off per year. You can still train more than that as long as it's cross-training in a different sport (such as swimming or biking if you play football).

Participating in more than one activity or sport can help athletes use different skills and avoid injury. Also, never exercise through pain. And, if you have an injury, make sure you give yourself enough time to heal. Your body—and your performance—will thank you.

Considering the benefits to the heart, muscles, joints, and mind, it's easy to see why exercise is wise. And the great thing about exercise is that it's never too late to start. Even small things can count as exercise when you're starting out—like taking a short bike ride, walking the dog, or raking leaves.

If you're already getting regular exercise now, try to keep it up after you graduate from high school. Staying fit is often one of the biggest challenges for people as they get busy with college and careers.

Chapter 50

Yoga

Yoga is a mind-body practice in complementary and alternative medicine (CAM) with origins in ancient Indian philosophy. The various styles of yoga that people use for health purposes typically combine physical postures, breathing techniques, and meditation or relaxation. This chapter provides a general overview of yoga.

Overview

Yoga, in its full form, combines physical postures, breathing exercises, meditation, and a distinct philosophy. Yoga is intended to increase relaxation and balance the mind, body, and the spirit.

Early written descriptions of yoga are in Sanskrit, the classical language of India. The word "yoga" comes from the Sanskrit word yuj, which means "yoke or union." It is believed that this describes the union between the mind and the body. The first known text, *The Yoga Sutras*, was written more than 2,000 years ago, although yoga may have been practiced as early as 5,000 years ago. Yoga was originally developed as a method of discipline and attitudes to help people reach spiritual enlightenment. The Sutras outline eight limbs or foundations of yoga practice that serve as spiritual guidelines:

1. *yama* (moral behavior)

2. *niyama* (healthy habits)

3. *asana* (physical postures)

About This Chapter: This chapter is excerpted from "Yoga For Health: An Introduction," National Center for Complementary and Alternative Medicine (www.nccam.nih.gov), June 2009.

4. *pranayama* (breathing exercises)

5. *pratyahara* (sense withdrawal)

6. *dharana* (concentration)

7. *dhyana* (contemplation)

8. *samadhi* (higher consciousness)

The numerous schools of yoga incorporate these eight limbs in varying proportions. Hatha yoga, the most commonly practiced in the United States and Europe, emphasizes two of the eight limbs: postures (asanas) and breathing exercises (pranayama). Some of the major styles of hatha yoga include Ananda, Anusara, Ashtanga, Bikram, Iyengar, Kripalu, Kundalini, and Viniyoga.

Use Of Yoga For Health In The United States

According to the 2007 National Health Interview Survey (NHIS), which included a comprehensive survey of CAM use by Americans, yoga is one of the top 10 CAM modalities used. More than 13 million adults had used yoga in the previous year, and between the 2002 and 2007 NHIS, use of yoga among adults increased by one percent (or approximately three million people). The 2007 survey also found that more than 1.5 million children used yoga in the previous year.

People use yoga for a variety of health conditions, including anxiety disorders or stress, asthma, high blood pressure, and depression. People also use yoga as part of a general health regimen—to achieve physical fitness and to relax.

The Status Of Yoga Research

Research suggests that yoga might:

• Improve mood and sense of well-being

• Counteract stress

• Reduce heart rate and blood pressure

• Increase lung capacity

• Improve muscle relaxation and body composition

• Help with conditions such as anxiety, depression, and insomnia

- Improve overall physical fitness, strength, and flexibility

- Positively affect levels of certain brain or blood chemicals

More well-designed studies are needed before definitive conclusions can be drawn about yoga's use for specific health conditions.

Side Effects And Risks

- Yoga is generally considered to be safe in healthy people when practiced appropriately. Studies have found it to be well tolerated, with few side effects.

- People with certain medical conditions should not use some yoga practices. For example, people with disc disease of the spine, extremely high or low blood pressure, glaucoma, retinal detachment, fragile or atherosclerotic arteries, a risk of blood clots, ear problems, severe osteoporosis, or cervical spondylitis should avoid some inverted poses.

- Although yoga during pregnancy is safe, if practiced under expert guidance, pregnant women should avoid certain poses that may be problematic.

Training, Licensing, And Certification

There are many training programs for yoga teachers throughout the country. These programs range from a few days to more than two years. Standards for teacher training and certification differ depending on the style of yoga.

If You Are Thinking About Yoga

- Do not use yoga as a replacement for conventional care or to postpone seeing a doctor about a medical problem.

- If you have a medical condition, consult with your health care provider before starting yoga.

- Ask about the physical demands of the type of yoga in which you are interested, as well as the training and experience of the yoga teacher you are considering.

- Look for published research studies on yoga for the health condition you are interested in.

- Tell your health care providers about any complementary and alternative practices you use. Give them a full picture of what you do to manage your health. This will help ensure coordinated and safe care.

There are organizations that register yoga teachers and training programs that have complied with minimum educational standards. For example, one nonprofit group requires at least 200 hours of training, with a specified number of hours in areas including techniques, teaching methodology, anatomy, physiology, and philosophy. However, there are currently no official or well-accepted licensing requirements for yoga teachers in the United States.

Chapter 51

Tai Chi

Tai chi, which originated in China as a martial art, is a mind-body practice in complementary and alternative medicine (CAM). Tai chi is sometimes referred to as "moving meditation" because practitioners move their bodies slowly, gently, and with awareness, while breathing deeply. This chapter provides a general overview of tai chi.

Overview

Tai chi developed in ancient China. It started as a martial art and a means of self-defense. Over time, people began to use it for health purposes, as well.

Accounts of the history of tai chi vary. A popular legend credits its origins to Chang San-Feng, a Taoist monk, who developed a set of 13 exercises that imitate the movements of animals. He also emphasized meditation and the concept of internal force (in contrast to the external force emphasized in other martial arts, such as kung fu and tae kwon do).

The term "tai chi" (shortened from "tai chi chuan") has been translated in various ways, such as "internal martial art" and "supreme ultimate fist." It is sometimes called "taiji" or "taijiquan."

Tai chi incorporates the Chinese concepts of yin and yang (opposing forces within the body) and qi (a vital energy or life force). Practicing tai chi is said to support a healthy balance of yin and yang, thereby aiding the flow of qi.

People practice tai chi by themselves or in groups. In the Chinese community, people commonly practice tai chi in nearby parks—often in early morning before going to work. There

About This Chapter: Information in this chapter is excerpted from "Tai Chi: An Introduction," National Center for Complementary and Alternative Medicine (www.nccam.nih.gov), August 2010.

Did You Know?

People practice tai chi for various health-related purposes, such as:

- For benefits associated with low-impact, weight-bearing, aerobic exercise
- To improve physical condition, muscle strength, coordination, and flexibility
- To improve balance and decrease the risk of falls, especially in elderly people
- To ease pain and stiffness—for example, from osteoarthritis
- To improve sleep
- For overall wellness

are many different styles, but all involve slow, relaxed, graceful movements, each flowing into the next. The body is in constant motion, and posture is important. The names of some of the movements evoke nature (for example, "Embrace Tiger, Return to Mountain"). Individuals practicing tai chi must also concentrate, putting aside distracting thoughts; and they must breathe in a deep and relaxed, but focused manner.

If You Are Thinking About Practicing Tai Chi

- Do not use tai chi as a replacement for conventional care or to postpone seeing a doctor about a medical problem.
- If you have a medical condition or have not exercised in a while, consult with your health care provider before starting tai chi.
- Keep in mind that learning tai chi from a video or book does not ensure that you are doing the movements correctly and safely.
- If you are considering a tai chi instructor, ask about the individual's training and experience.
- Look for published research studies on tai chi for the health condition you are interested in.
- Tell all your health care providers about any complementary and alternative practices you use. Give them a full picture of what you do to manage your health. This will help ensure coordinated and safe care.

Side Effects And Risks

Tai chi is a relatively safe practice. However, there are some cautions:

- As with any exercise regimen, if you overdo practice, you may have sore muscles or sprains.

- Tai chi instructors often recommend that you do not practice tai chi right after a meal, or when you are very tired, or if you have an active infection.

- If you are pregnant, or if you have a hernia, joint problems, back pain, fractures, or severe osteoporosis, your health care provider may advise you to modify or avoid certain postures in tai chi.

Training, Licensing, And Certification

Tai chi instructors do not have to be licensed, and the practice is not regulated by the Federal Government or individual states. In traditional tai chi instruction, a student learns from a master teacher. To become an instructor, an experienced student of tai chi must obtain a master teacher's approval. Currently, training programs vary. Some training programs award certificates; some offer weekend workshops. There is no standard training for instructors.

Chapter 52

Use Your Senses To Relieve Stress

There are countless techniques for preventing stress. Yoga and meditation work wonders for improving our coping skills. But who can take a moment to chant or meditate during school, a job interview, or a disagreement? For these situations, you need something more immediate and accessible. That's when quick stress relief comes to the rescue.

The speediest way to stamp out stress is by engaging one or more of your senses—your sense of sight, sound, taste, smell, touch, or movement—to rapidly calm and energize yourself.

Remember exploring your senses in elementary school? Adolescents can take a tip from grade school lessons by revisiting the senses and learning how they can help us prevent stress overload. Use the following exercises to identify the types of stress-busting sensory experiences that work quickly and effectively for you.

Sights

If you're a visual person, try to manage and relieve stress by surrounding yourself with soothing and uplifting images. You can also try closing your eyes and imagining the soothing images. Here are a few visually-based activities that may work as quick stress relievers:

- Look at a cherished photo or a favorite memento.

- Bring the outside indoors; buy a plant or some flowers to enliven your space.

- Enjoy the beauty of nature–a garden, the beach, a park, or your own backyard.

About This Chapter: Information in this chapter is from "The Basics of Quick Stress Relief: Engage Your Senses," U.S. Department of Veterans Affairs, Phoenix VA Health Care System (www.pheonix.va.gov), December 2011.

- Surround yourself with colors that lift your spirits.

- Close your eyes and picture a situation or place that feels peaceful and rejuvenating.

Sound

Are you sensitive to sounds and noises? Are you a music lover? If so, stress-relieving exercises that focus on your auditory sense may work particularly well. Experiment with the following sounds, noting how quickly your stress levels drop as you listen.

- Sing or hum a favorite tune. Listen to uplifting music.

- Tune in to the soundtrack of nature—crashing waves, the wind rustling the trees, birds singing.

- Buy a small fountain, so you can enjoy the soothing sound of running water.

- Hang wind chimes near an open window.

Smell And Scents

If you tend to zone out or freeze when stressed, surround yourself with smells that are energizing and invigorating. If you tend to become overly agitated under stress, look for scents that are comforting and calming.

- Light a scented candle or burn some incense.

- Lie down in sheets scented with lavender.

- Smell the roses—or another type of flower.

- Enjoy the clean, fresh air in the great outdoors.

- Spritz on your favorite perfume or cologne.

Touch

Experiment with your sense of touch, playing with different tactile sensations. Focus on things you can feel that are relaxing and renewing. Use the following suggestions as a jumping off point:

- Wrap yourself in a warm blanket.

- Pet a dog or cat.

- Hold a comforting object (a stuffed animal, a favorite memento).

- Soak in a hot bath.

- Give yourself a hand or neck massage.

- Wear clothing that feels soft against your skin.

Taste

Slowly savoring a favorite treat can be very relaxing, but mindless stress eating will only add to your stress and your waistline. The key is to indulge your sense of taste mindfully and in moderation. Eat slowly, focusing on the feel of the food in your mouth and the taste on your tongue:

- Chew a piece of sugarless gum.

- Indulge in a small piece of dark chocolate.

- Sip a steaming cup of coffee or tea or a refreshing cold drink.

- Eat a perfectly ripe piece of fruit.

- Enjoy a healthy, crunchy snack (celery, carrots, or trail mix).

Movement

If you tend to shut down when you're under stress, stress-relieving activities that get you moving may be particularly helpful. Anything that engages the muscles or gets you up and active can work. Here are a few suggestions:

- Run in place or jump up and down.

- Dance around.

- Stretch or roll your head in circles.

- Go for a short walk.

- Squeeze a rubbery stress ball.

The Power Of Imagination

Sensory rich memories can also quickly reduce stress. After drawing upon your sensory toolbox becomes habit, another approach is to learn to simply imagine vivid sensations when stress strikes. Believe it or not, the mere memory of your baby's face will have the same calming or energizing effects on your brain as seeing her photo. So if you can recall a strong sensation, you'll never be without access to your quick stress relief toolbox.

Chapter 53

Meditation

Meditation is a mind-body practice in complementary and alternative medicine (CAM). There are many types of meditation, most of which originated in ancient religious and spiritual traditions. Generally, a person who is meditating uses certain techniques, such as a specific posture, focused attention, and an open attitude toward distractions. Meditation may be practiced for many reasons, such as to increase calmness and physical relaxation, to improve psychological balance, to cope with illness, or to enhance overall health and well-being. This chapter provides a general introduction to meditation.

Overview

The term meditation refers to a group of techniques, such as mantra meditation, relaxation response, mindfulness meditation, and Zen Buddhist meditation. Most meditative techniques started in Eastern religious or spiritual traditions. These techniques have been used by many different cultures throughout the world for thousands of years. Today, many people use meditation outside of its traditional religious or cultural settings, for health and well-being.

In meditation, a person learns to focus attention. Some forms of meditation instruct the practitioner to become mindful of thoughts, feelings, and sensations and to observe them in a nonjudgmental way. This practice is believed to result in a state of greater calmness and physical relaxation, and psychological balance. Practicing meditation can change how a person relates to the flow of emotions and thoughts.

Most types of meditation have four elements in common:

About This Chapter: Information in this chapter is excerpted from "Meditation: An Introduction," National Center for Complementary and Alternative Medicine (www.nccam.nih.gov), June 2010.

- **Quiet Location:** Meditation is usually practiced in a quiet place with as few distractions as possible. This can be particularly helpful for beginners.

- **Specific, Comfortable Posture:** Depending on the type being practiced, meditation can be done while sitting, lying down, standing, walking, or in other positions.

- **Focus Of Attention:** Focusing one's attention is usually a part of meditation. For example, the meditator may focus on a mantra (a specially chosen word or set of words), an object, or the sensations of the breath. Some forms of meditation involve paying attention to whatever is the dominant content of consciousness.

- **Open Attitude:** Having an open attitude during meditation means letting distractions come and go naturally without judging them. When the attention goes to distracting or wandering thoughts, they are not suppressed; instead, the meditator gently brings attention back to the focus. In some types of meditation, the meditator learns to "observe" thoughts and emotions while meditating.

Meditation used as CAM is a type of mind-body medicine. Generally, mind-body medicine focuses on:

- Interactions among the brain/mind, the rest of the body, and behavior

- Ways in which emotional, mental, social, spiritual, and behavioral factors can directly affect health

Uses Of Meditation For Health In The United States

A 2007 national Government survey that asked about CAM use in a sample of 23,393 U.S. adults found that 9.4 percent of respondents (representing more than 20 million people) had used meditation in the past 12 months—compared with 7.6 percent of respondents (representing more than 15 million people) in a similar survey conducted in 2002. The 2007 survey also asked about CAM use in a sample of 9,417 children; one percent (representing 725,000 children) had used meditation in the past 12 months.

People use meditation for various health problems, such as:

- Anxiety

- Pain

- Depression

- Stress

- Insomnia

- Physical or emotional symptoms that may be associated with chronic illnesses (such as heart disease, HIV/AIDS, and cancer) and their treatment

Meditation is also used for overall wellness.

Examples Of Meditation Practices

Mindfulness meditation and transcendental meditation (also known as TM) are two common forms of meditation. The National Center for Complementary and Alternative Medicine (NCCAM) sponsored research projects are studying both types of meditation.

Mindfulness meditation is an essential component of Buddhism. In one common form of mindfulness meditation, the meditator is taught to bring attention to the sensation of the flow of the breath in and out of the body. The meditator learns to focus attention on what is being experienced, without reacting to or judging it. This is seen as helping the meditator learn to experience thoughts and emotions in normal daily life with greater balance and acceptance.

The TM technique is derived from Hindu traditions. It uses a mantra (a word, sound, or phrase repeated silently) to prevent distracting thoughts from entering the mind. The goal of TM is to achieve a state of relaxed awareness.

How Meditation Might Work

Practicing meditation has been shown to induce some changes in the body. By learning more about what goes on in the body during meditation, researchers hope to be able to identify diseases or conditions for which meditation might be useful.

Some types of meditation might work by affecting the autonomic (involuntary) nervous system. This system regulates many organs and muscles, controlling functions such as heartbeat, sweating, breathing, and digestion. It has two major parts:

- The sympathetic nervous system helps mobilize the body for action. When a person is under stress, it produces the "fight-or-flight response" where the heart rate and breathing rate go up and blood vessels narrow (restricting the flow of blood).

- The parasympathetic nervous system causes the heart rate and breathing rate to slow down, the blood vessels to dilate (improving blood flow), and the flow of digestive juices increases.

It is thought that some types of meditation might work by reducing activity in the sympathetic nervous system and increasing activity in the parasympathetic nervous system.

Mindfulness Meditation And Structural Changes In The Brain

According to a recent study, practicing mindfulness meditation appears to be associated with measurable changes in the brain regions involved in memory, learning, and emotion. Mindfulness meditation focuses attention on breathing to develop increased awareness of the present. Previous research has demonstrated that mindfulness mediation may reduce symptoms of anxiety, depression, and chronic pain, but little is known about its effects on the brain. The focus of the current study—published in the journal *Psychiatry Research: Neuroimaging*—was to identify brain regions that changed in participants enrolled in an 8-week mindfulness-based stress reduction program.

In this study, researchers from Massachusetts General Hospital, Bender Institute of Neuroimaging in Germany, and the University of Massachusetts Medical School, took magnetic resonance images of the brains of 16 participants 2 weeks before and after they joined the meditation program. (Participants were physician- and self-referred individuals seeking stress reduction.) Researchers also took brain images of a control group of 17 non-meditators over a similar time period. Participants in the meditation group attended weekly sessions that included mindfulness training exercises and received audio recordings for guided meditation practice at home. They also kept track of how much time they practiced each day. Members of both groups completed a questionnaire, before and after joining the group, which measured five aspects of mindfulness: observing, describing, acting with awareness, non-judging of inner experience, and non-reactivity to inner experience.

Brain images in the meditation group revealed increases in gray matter concentration in the left hippocampus. The hippocampus is an area of the brain involved in learning, memory, and emotional control, and is suspected of playing a role in producing some of the positive effects of meditation. Gray matter also increased in four other brain regions (though not in the insula, a region that has shown changes in other meditation studies) in the meditation group. Responses to the questionnaire indicated improvements in three of the five aspects of mindfulness in the mediators, but not the control group.

The researchers concluded that these findings may represent an underlying brain mechanism associated with mindfulness-based improvements in mental health. Additional studies are needed to determine the associations between specific types of brain change and behavioral mechanisms thought to improve a variety of disorders.

Source: "Mindfulness Meditation Is Associated With Structural Changes In The Brain," National Center for Complementary and Alternative Medicine (www.nccam.gov), January 2011.

In one area of research, scientists are using sophisticated tools to determine whether meditation is associated with significant changes in brain function. A number of researchers believe that these changes account for many of meditation's effects.

It is also possible that practicing meditation may work by improving the mind's ability to pay attention. Since attention is involved in performing everyday tasks and regulating mood, meditation might lead to other benefits.

A 2007 NCCAM-funded review of the scientific literature found some evidence suggesting that meditation is associated with potentially beneficial health effects. However, the overall evidence was inconclusive. The reviewers concluded that future research needs to be more rigorous before firm conclusions can be drawn.

Side Effects And Risks

Meditation is considered to be safe for healthy people. There have been rare reports that meditation could cause or worsen symptoms in people who have certain psychiatric problems, but this question has not been fully researched. People with physical limitations may not be able to participate in certain meditative practices involving physical movement. Individuals with existing mental or physical health conditions should speak with their health care providers prior to starting a meditative practice and make their meditation instructor aware of their condition.

If You Are Thinking About Using Meditation Practices

- Do not use meditation as a replacement for conventional care or as a reason to postpone seeing a doctor about a medical problem.

- Ask about the training and experience of the meditation instructor you are considering.

- Look for published research studies on meditation for the health condition in which you are interested.

- Tell all your health care providers about any complementary and alternative practices you use. Give them a full picture of what you do to manage your health. This will help ensure coordinated and safe care.

Chapter 54

Relaxation Techniques

Relaxation techniques include a number of practices such as progressive relaxation, guided imagery, biofeedback, self-hypnosis, and deep breathing exercises. The goal is similar in all: to consciously produce the body's natural relaxation response, characterized by slower breathing, lower blood pressure, and a feeling of calm and well-being.

Relaxation techniques (also called relaxation response techniques) may be used by some to release tension and to counteract the ill effects of stress. Relaxation techniques are also used to induce sleep, reduce pain, and calm emotions. This chapter provides a general overview of relaxation techniques.

About Relaxation Techniques

Relaxation is more than a state of mind; it physically changes the way your body functions. When your body is relaxed breathing slows, blood pressure and oxygen consumption decrease, and some people report an increased sense of well-being. This is called the "relaxation response." Being able to produce the relaxation response using relaxation techniques may counteract the effects of long-term stress, which may contribute to, or worsen, a range of health problems including depression, digestive disorders, headaches, high blood pressure, and insomnia.

Relaxation techniques often combine breathing and focused attention on pleasing thoughts and images to calm the mind and the body. Most methods require only brief instruction from a

About This Chapter: Information in this chapter is excerpted from "Relaxation Techniques For Health: An Introduction," National Center for Complementary and Alternative Medicine (www.nccam.nih.gov), August 2011.

book or experienced practitioner before they can be done without assistance. These techniques may be most effective when practiced regularly and combined with good nutrition, regular exercise, and a strong social support system.

- **Autogenic Training:** When using this method, you focus on the physical sensation of your own breathing or heartbeat and picture your body as warm, heavy, and/or relaxed.

- **Biofeedback:** Biofeedback-assisted relaxation uses electronic devices to teach you how to consciously produce the relaxation response. Biofeedback is sometimes used to relieve conditions that are caused or worsened by stress.

- **Deep Breathing Or Breathing Exercises:** To relax using this method, you consciously slow your breathing and focus on taking regular and deep breaths.

- **Guided Imagery:** For this technique, you focus on pleasant images to replace negative or stressful feelings and relax. Guided imagery may be directed by you or a practitioner through storytelling or descriptions designed to suggest mental images (also called visualization).

- **Progressive Relaxation:** Also called Jacobson's progressive relaxation or progressive muscle relaxation, for this relaxation method, you focus on tightening and relaxing each muscle group. Progressive relaxation is often combined with guided imagery and breathing exercises.

- **Self-Hypnosis:** In self-hypnosis, you produce the relaxation response with a phrase or nonverbal cue (called a "suggestion"). Self-hypnosis may be used to relieve pain (tension headaches, labor, or minor surgery) as well as to treat anxiety and irritable bowel syndrome.

Mind and body practices, such as meditation and yoga are also sometimes considered relaxation techniques.

Use Of Relaxation Techniques For Health In The United States

People may use relaxation techniques as part of a comprehensive plan to treat, prevent, or reduce symptoms of a variety of conditions including stress, high blood pressure, chronic pain, insomnia, depression, labor pain, headache, cardiovascular disease, anxiety, chemotherapy side effects, and others. Most of those people reported using a book to learn the techniques rather than seeing a practitioner.

How Relaxation Techniques May Work

To understand how consciously producing the relaxation response may affect your health, it is helpful to understand how your body responds to the opposite of relaxation—stress.

When you are under stress, your body releases hormones that produce the "fight-or-flight response," which means your heart rate and breathing rate go up and blood vessels narrow (restricting the flow of blood). This response allows energy to flow to parts of your body that need to take action, for example the muscles and the heart. However useful this response may be in the short term, there is evidence that when your body remains in a stress state for a long time, emotional or physical damage can occur. Long-term or chronic stress (lasting months or years) may reduce your body's ability to fight off illness and lead to or worsen certain health conditions. Chronic stress may lead to high blood pressure, headaches, stomach ache, and other symptoms. Stress may worsen certain conditions, such as asthma. Stress also has been linked to depression, anxiety, and other mental illnesses.

In contrast to the stress response, the relaxation response slows the heart rate, lowers blood pressure, and decreases oxygen consumption and levels of stress hormones. Because relaxation is the opposite of stress, the theory is that voluntarily creating the relaxation response through regular use of relaxation techniques could counteract the negative effects of stress.

Status Of Research On Relaxation Techniques

In the past 30 years, there has been considerable interest in the relaxation response and how inducing this state may benefit health. Research has focused primarily on illness and conditions in which stress may play a role either as the cause of the condition or as a factor that can make the condition worse.

Currently, there is some evidence that relaxation techniques may be an effective part of an overall treatment plan for some disorders, including:

- **Anxiety:** Studies have suggested that relaxation may assist in the treatment of phobias or panic disorder. Relaxation techniques have also been used to relieve anxiety for people in stressful situations, such as when undergoing a medical procedure.

- **Depression:** In 2008, a major review of the evidence for relaxation in the treatment of depression found that relaxation techniques were more effective than no treatment for depression, but not as effective as cognitive-behavioral therapy.

- **Headache:** There is some evidence that biofeedback and other relaxation techniques may be helpful for relieving tension or migraine headaches. In some cases, these mind and body techniques were more effective than medications for reducing the frequency, intensity, and severity of headaches.

- **Pain:** Some studies have shown that relaxation techniques may help reduce abdominal and surgery pain.

The results of research on relaxation to promote overall health or well-being or to treat other health conditions have been mixed or unclear. These conditions include:

- **High Blood Pressure:** A 2008 review of evidence for relaxation in the treatment of high blood pressure found some evidence that progressive muscle relaxation lowered blood pressure a small amount. However, the review found no evidence that this effect was enough to reduce the risk of heart disease, stroke, or other health issues due to high blood pressure. In a recent randomized controlled trial, eight weeks of relaxation response/stress management was shown to reduce systolic blood pressure in hypertensive older adults, and some patients were able to reduce hypertension medication without an increase in blood pressure.

- **Asthma:** Several reviews of the literature have suggested that relaxation techniques, including guided imagery, may temporarily help improve lung function and quality of life and relieve anxiety in people with asthma. A more recent randomized clinical trial of asthma found that relaxation techniques may help improve immune function. More studies are needed to confirm this finding.

- **Nausea:** Relaxation techniques may help relieve nausea caused by chemotherapy.

- **Fibromyalgia:** Although some preliminary studies report that using relaxation or guided imagery techniques may sometimes improve pain and reduce fatigue from fibromyalgia, more research is needed.

- **Irritable Bowel Syndrome (IBS):** Some studies have indicated that relaxation techniques may prevent or relieve symptoms of IBS in some participants. One review of the research found some evidence that self-hypnosis may be useful in the treatment of IBS.

- **Heart Disease And Heart Symptoms:** Researchers have looked at relaxation techniques for the treatment of angina and the prevention of heart disease. When a cardiac rehabilitation program was combined with relaxation response training in a clinic, participants experienced significant reductions in blood pressure, decreases in lipid levels, and increases in psychological functioning when compared to participants' status before the program. Although studies have shown that relaxation techniques combined with other lifestyle changes and standard medical care may reduce the risk of recurrent heart attack, more study is needed.

- **Insomnia:** There is some evidence that relaxation techniques can help in treating chronic insomnia.

Researchers have found some evidence on the effectiveness of relaxation techniques for:

- **Temporomandibular Disorder (TMD):** TMD causes pain and loss of motion in the jaw joints. A review of the literature found that relaxation techniques and biofeedback were more effective than placebo in decreasing pain and increasing jaw function.
- **Ringing In The Ears:** Use of relaxation exercises may help patients cope with the condition.
- **Smoking Cessation:** Relaxation exercises may help reduce the desire to smoke.
- **Overactive Bladder:** Bladder retraining combined with relaxation and other exercises may help control urinary urgency.
- **Nightmares:** Relaxation exercises may be effective in treating nightmares of unknown cause and those associated with posttraumatic stress disorder.
- **Hot Flashes:** Relaxation exercises involving slow, controlled deep breathing may help relieve hot flashes associated with menopause.

Researchers have found no significant change in outcomes from relaxation techniques used during cardiac catheterization. However, patients experienced less distress prior to the procedure. Future research may investigate whether this has any long-term effect on outlook and recovery.

Many of the studies of relaxation therapy and health have followed a small number of patients for weeks or months. Longer studies involving more participants may reveal more about the cumulative effects of using relaxation techniques regularly.

Side Effects And Risks

Relaxation techniques are generally considered safe for healthy people. There have been rare reports that certain relaxation techniques might cause or worsen symptoms in people with epilepsy or certain psychiatric conditions, or with a history of abuse or trauma. People with heart disease should talk to their doctor before doing progressive muscle relaxation.

Relaxation techniques are often used as part of a treatment plan and not as the sole treatment for potentially serious health conditions.

Training, Licensing, And Certification

There is no formal credential or license required for practicing or teaching most relaxation techniques. However, the techniques may be used or taught by licensed professionals, including physicians, recreational therapists, and psychologists.

If You Are Thinking About Using Relaxation Techniques For Health

- Do not use relaxation techniques as a replacement for conventional care or to postpone seeing a doctor about a medical problem.
- Ask about the training and experience of the practitioner or instructor you are considering for any complementary and alternative medicine (CAM) practice.
- Look for published research studies on relaxation for the health condition in which you are interested. Remember that some claims for using relaxation therapies may exceed the available scientific evidence.
- Tell all your health care providers about any complementary and alternative practices you use. Give them a full picture of what you do to manage your health. This will help ensure coordinated and safe care.

Chapter 55

Massage Therapy

Massage therapy has a long history in cultures around the world. Today, people use many different types of massage therapy for a variety of health-related purposes. In the United States, massage therapy is often considered part of complementary and alternative medicine (CAM), although it does have some conventional uses. This chapter provides a general overview of massage therapy.

History Of Massage

Massage therapy dates back thousands of years. References to massage appear in writings from ancient China, Japan, India, Arabic nations, Egypt, Greece (Hippocrates defined medicine as "the art of rubbing"), and Rome.

Massage became widely used in Europe during the Renaissance. In the 1850s, two American physicians who had studied in Sweden introduced massage therapy in the United States, where it became popular and was promoted for a variety of health purposes. With scientific and technological advances in medical treatment during the 1930s and 1940s, massage fell out of favor in the United States. Interest in massage revived in the 1970s, especially among athletes.

Use Of Massage Therapy In The United States

According to the 2007 National Health Interview Survey, which included a comprehensive survey of CAM use by Americans, an estimated 18 million U.S. adults and 700,000 children had received massage therapy in the previous year.

About This Chapter: Information in this chapter is excerpted from "Massage Therapy: An Introduction," National Center for Complementary and Alternative Medicine (www.nccam.nih.gov), August 2010.

People use massage for a variety of health-related purposes, including to relieve pain, rehabilitate sports injuries, reduce stress, increase relaxation, address anxiety and depression, and aid general wellness.

Defining Massage Therapy

The term "massage therapy" encompasses many different techniques. In general, therapists press, rub, and otherwise manipulate the muscles and other soft tissues of the body. They most often use their hands and fingers, but may use their forearms, elbows, or feet.

The Practice Of Massage Therapy

Massage therapists work in a variety of settings, including private offices, hospitals, nursing homes, studios, and sport and fitness facilities. Some also travel to patients' homes or workplaces. They usually try to provide a calm, soothing environment.

Therapists usually ask new patients about symptoms, medical history, and desired results. They may also perform an evaluation through touch, to locate painful or tense areas and determine how much pressure to apply.

Typically, the patient lies on a table, either in loose-fitting clothing or undressed (covered with a sheet, except for the area being massaged). The therapist may use oil or lotion to reduce friction on the skin. Sometimes, people receive massage therapy while sitting in a chair. A massage session may be fairly brief, but may also last an hour or even longer.

Research Status

Although scientific research on massage therapy—whether it works and, if so, how—is limited, there is evidence that massage may benefit some patients. Conclusions generally cannot yet be drawn about its effectiveness for specific health conditions.

According to one analysis, however, research supports the general conclusion that massage therapy is effective. The studies included in the analysis suggest that a single session of massage therapy can reduce "state anxiety" (a reaction to a particular situation), blood pressure, and heart rate; and multiple sessions can reduce "trait anxiety" (general anxiety-proneness), depression, and pain. In addition, recent studies suggest that massage may benefit certain conditions, for example:

- A 2008 review of 13 clinical trials found evidence that massage might be useful for chronic low-back pain. Clinical practice guidelines issued in 2007 by the American Pain Society and the American College of Physicians recommend that physicians consider using certain CAM therapies, including massage (as well as acupuncture, chiropractic, progressive relaxation, and yoga), when patients with chronic low-back pain do not respond to conventional treatment.

- A multisite study of more than 300 hospice patients with advanced cancer concluded that massage may help to relieve pain and improve mood for these patients.

- A study of 64 patients with chronic neck pain found that therapeutic massage was more beneficial than a self-care book, in terms of improving function and relieving symptoms.

There are numerous theories about how massage therapy may affect the body. For example, the "gate control theory" suggests that massage may provide stimulation that helps to block pain signals sent to the brain. Other theories suggest that massage might stimulate the release of certain chemicals in the body, such as serotonin or endorphins, or cause beneficial mechanical changes in the body. However, additional studies are needed to test the various theories.

Safety

Massage therapy appears to have few serious risks—if it is performed by a properly trained therapist and if appropriate cautions are followed. The number of serious injuries reported is very small. Side effects of massage therapy may include temporary pain or discomfort, bruising, swelling, and a sensitivity or allergy to massage oils.

Cautions about massage therapy include the following:

- Vigorous massage should be avoided by people with bleeding disorders or low blood platelet counts, and by people taking blood-thinning medications such as warfarin.

- Massage should not be done in any area of the body with blood clots, fractures, open or healing wounds, skin infections, or weakened bones (such as from osteoporosis or cancer), or where there has been a recent surgery.

Types Of Massage Therapy: A Few Examples

In Swedish massage, the therapist uses long strokes, kneading, deep circular movements, vibration, and tapping. Sports massage is similar to Swedish massage, adapted specifically to the needs of athletes. Among the many other examples are deep tissue massage and trigger point massage, which focuses on myofascial trigger points—muscle "knots" that are painful when pressed and can cause symptoms elsewhere in the body.

- Although massage therapy appears to be generally safe for cancer patients, they should consult their oncologist before having a massage that involves deep or intense pressure. Any direct pressure over a tumor usually is discouraged. Cancer patients should discuss any concerns about massage therapy with their oncologist.

- Pregnant women should consult their health care provider before using massage therapy.

Training, Licensing, And Certification

There are approximately 1,500 massage therapy schools and training programs in the United States. In addition to hands-on practice of massage techniques, students generally learn about the body and how it works, business practices, and ethics. Massage training programs generally are approved by a state board. Some may also be accredited by an independent agency, such as the Commission on Massage Therapy Accreditation (COMTA).

As of 2010, 43 states and the District of Columbia had laws regulating massage therapy. In some states, regulation is by town ordinance.

The National Certification Board for Therapeutic Massage and Bodywork certifies practitioners who pass a national examination. Increasingly, states that license massage therapists require

If You Are Thinking About Using Massage Therapy

- Do not use massage therapy to replace your regular medical care or as a reason to postpone seeing a health care provider about a medical problem.

- If you have a medical condition and are unsure whether massage therapy would be appropriate for you, discuss your concerns with your health care provider. Your health care provider may also be able to help you select a massage therapist. You might also look for published research articles on massage therapy for your condition.

- Before deciding to begin massage therapy, ask about the therapist's training, experience, and credentials. Also ask about the number of treatments that might be needed, the cost, and insurance coverage.

- If a massage therapist suggests using other CAM practices (for example, herbs or other supplements, or a special diet), discuss it first with your regular health care provider.

- Tell all your health care providers about any complementary and alternative practices you use. Give them a full picture of what you do to manage your health. This will ensure coordinated and safe care.

them to have a minimum of 500 hours of training at an accredited institution, pass a national exam, meet specific continuing education requirements, and carry malpractice insurance.

In addition to massage therapists, health care providers such as chiropractors and physical therapists may have training in massage.

Licenses And Certifications

Some common licenses or certifications for massage therapists include:

- LMT: Licensed Massage Therapist

- LMP: Licensed Massage Practitioner

- CMT: Certified Massage Therapist

- NCTMB: Has met the credentialing requirements (including passing an exam) of the National Certification Board for Therapeutic Massage and Bodywork, for practicing therapeutic massage and bodywork

- NCTM: Has met the credentialing requirements (including passing an exam) of the National Certification Board for Therapeutic Massage and Bodywork, for practicing therapeutic massage

Chapter 56

Spirituality

What is spirituality?

Spirituality has been defined in numerous ways. These include: a belief in a power operating in the universe that is greater than oneself, a sense of interconnectedness with all living creatures, and an awareness of the purpose and meaning of life and the development of personal, absolute values. It's the way you find meaning, hope, comfort, and inner peace in your life. Although spirituality is often associated with religious life, many believe that personal spirituality can be developed outside of religion. Acts of compassion and selflessness, altruism, and the experience of inner peace are all characteristics of spirituality. Many Americans are becoming interested in the role of spirituality in their health and health care. This may be because of dissatisfaction with the impersonal nature of our current medical system, and the realization that medical science does not have answers to every question about health and wellness.

What is the history of spirituality and health care?

In most healing traditions and through generations of healers in the early beginnings of Western medicine, concerns of the body and spirit were intertwined. But with the coming of the scientific revolution and the enlightenment, these considerations were removed from the medical system. Today, however, a growing number of studies reveal that spirituality may play a bigger role in the healing process than the medical community previously thought.

How does spirituality influence health?

Spiritual practices tend to improve coping skills and social support, foster feelings of optimism and hope, promote healthy behavior, reduce feelings of depression and anxiety, and encourage a sense of relaxation. By alleviating stressful feelings and promoting healing ones, spirituality can positively influence immune, cardiovascular (heart and blood vessels), hormonal, and nervous systems. An example of a religion that promotes a healthy lifestyle is Seventh Day Adventists. Those who follow this religion, a particularly healthy population, are instructed by their Church not to consume alcohol, eat pork, or smoke tobacco. In a 10 year study of Seventh Day Adventists in the Netherlands, researchers found that Adventist men lived 8.9 years longer than the national average, and Adventist women lived 3.6 years longer. For both men and women, the chance of dying from cancer or heart disease was 60–66% less, respectively, than the national average.

Again, the health benefits of religion and spirituality do not stem solely from healthy lifestyles. Many researchers believe that certain beliefs, attitudes, and practices associated with being a spiritual person influence health. In a recent study of people with acquired immune deficiency syndrome (AIDS), those who had faith in God, compassion toward others, a sense of inner peace, and were religious had a better chance of surviving for a long time than those who did not live with such belief systems. Qualities like faith, hope, and forgiveness, and the use of social support and prayer seem to have a noticeable effect on health and healing.

- **Faith:** A person's most deeply held beliefs strongly influence his or her health. Some researchers believe that faith increases the body's resistance to stress. In a 1988 clinical study of women undergoing breast biopsies, the women with the lowest stress hormone levels were those who used their faith and prayer to cope with stress.

- **Hope:** Without hope—a positive attitude that a person assumes in the face of difficulty—many people become depressed and prone to illness. In a 35 year clinical study of Harvard graduates, researchers found that those graduates who expressed hope and optimism lived longer and had fewer illnesses in their lifetime.

- **Forgiveness:** A practice that is encouraged by many spiritual and religious traditions, forgiveness is a release of hostility and resentment from past hurts. In 1997, a Stanford University study found that college students trained to forgive someone who had hurt them were significantly less angry, more hopeful, and better able to deal with emotions than students not trained to forgive. Another survey of 1,400 adults found that willingness to forgive oneself, and others, and the feeling that one is forgiven by God, have beneficial health effects. Some researchers suggest that emotions like anger and resentment cause stress hormones to accumulate in the blood, and that forgiveness reduces this build up.

- **Love And Social Support:** A close network of family and friends that lends help and emotional support has been found to offer protection against many diseases. Researchers believe that people who experience love and support tend to resist unhealthy behaviors and feel less stressed. In a clinical study of a close knit Italian American community in Pennsylvania, researchers found that the death rate from heart attack was half that of the United States' average. Researchers concluded that the strong social support network helped protect this population from heart disease.

- **Prayer:** The act of putting oneself in the presence of or conversing with a higher power has been used as a means of healing across all cultures throughout the ages. Today, many Americans believe that prayer is an important part of daily life. In a 1996 poll, one half of doctors reported that they believe prayer helps patients, and 67% reported praying for a patient. Researchers are also studying intercessory prayer (asking a higher power to intervene on behalf of another either known or unknown to the person praying; also called distance prayer or distance healing). Although it is particularly difficult to study the effect of distance prayer, current research in coronary care units (intensive care units in hospitals devoted to people with severe heart disease, like those who just suffered a heart attack) suggests that there is benefit. Compared to those who were not prayed for, patients who were prayed for showed general improvements in the course of their illness, less complications, and even fewer deaths.

What illnesses and conditions respond well to spirituality?

Programs with a strong spiritual component, such as Alcoholics Anonymous (AA), show that spiritual disciplines may be especially effective for drug and alcohol addiction. The regular practice of prayer and meditation is strongly associated with recovery and abstinence from drugs.

Results from several studies indicate that people with strong religious and spiritual beliefs heal faster from surgery, are less anxious and depressed, have lower blood pressure, and cope better with chronic illnesses such as arthritis, diabetes, heart disease, cancer, and spinal cord injury.

One clinical study at Duke University found that people who attend regular religious services tend to have better immune function. In another clinical study of 232 older adults undergoing heart surgery, those who were religious were three times less likely to die within the six months after surgery than those who were not. Not one of the 37 people in this study who described themselves as deeply religious died. Of course, the studies are not comprehensive, and many people find help in spiritual resources for numerous conditions.

Can spirituality have a negative impact on health?

Some experts warn that religious beliefs can be harmful when they encourage excessive guilt, fear, and lowered self-worth. Similarly, physicians should avoid advocating for particular spiritual practices; this can be inappropriate, intrusive, and induce a feeling of guilt or even harm if the implication is that ill health is a result of insufficient faith. It is also important to note that spirituality does not guarantee health. Finally, there is the risk that people may substitute prayer for medical care or that spiritual practice could delay the receipt of necessary medical treatment.

How can I receive spiritual counseling when I am in the hospital?

Many hospitals have access to counselors from organized religions. If you would like spiritual counseling or someone to pray with, ask your doctor to refer a counselor.

What is the future of spirituality in medical practice?

Many medical schools in the United States have included spiritual teachings in their curricula. However, what role, if any, a doctor should play in assisting or guiding patients in spiritual matters remains controversial. In addition, given that there appears to be a growing belief in the connection between spirituality and health, scientists in this field feel that research should begin to focus on assessing the validity of this connection, a better understanding of why there is this connection, and how it works. There is also interesting research emerging that evaluates the impact of religion and spirituality (both the child's and the parents') on the health of children and adolescents.

Chapter 57

Laughter

Humor is infectious. The sound of roaring laughter is far more contagious than any cough, sniffle, or sneeze. When laughter is shared, it binds people together and increases happiness and intimacy. Laughter also triggers healthy physical changes in the body. Humor and laughter strengthen your immune system, boost your energy, diminish pain, and protect you from the damaging effects of stress. Best of all, this priceless medicine is fun, free, and easy to use.

Laughter Is Strong Medicine For Mind And Body

Laughter is a powerful antidote to stress, pain, and conflict. Nothing works faster or more dependably to bring your mind and body back into balance than a good laugh. Humor lightens your burdens, inspires hopes, connects you to others, and keeps you grounded, focused, and alert.

With so much power to heal and renew, the ability to laugh easily and frequently is a tremendous resource for surmounting problems, enhancing your relationships, and supporting both physical and emotional health.

Laughter Is Good For Your Health

- **Laughter relaxes the whole body.** A good, hearty laugh relieves physical tension and stress, leaving your muscles relaxed for up to 45 minutes after.

About This Chapter: "Laughter is the Best Medicine," by Melinda Smith, M.A., Gina Kemp, M.A., and Jeanne Segal, Ph.D., updated March 2013. © 2013 Helpguide.org. All rights reserved. Reprinted with permission. Helpguide provides a detailed list of references and resources for this article, with links to related Helpguide topics and information from other websites. For a complete list of these resources, go to http://www.helpguide.org/life/humor_laughter_health.htm.

> "Your sense of humor is one of the most powerful tools you have to make certain that your daily mood and emotional state support good health."
>
> —Paul E. McGhee, PhD

- **Laughter boosts the immune system.** Laughter decreases stress hormones and increases immune cells and infection-fighting antibodies, thus improving your resistance to disease.

- **Laughter triggers the release of endorphins.** The body's natural feel-good chemicals, endorphins, promote an overall sense of well-being and can even temporarily relieve pain.

- **Laughter protects the heart.** Laughter improves the function of blood vessels and increases blood flow, which can help protect you against a heart attack and other cardiovascular problems.

The Benefits Of Laughter

Physical Health Benefits

- Boosts immunity
- Decreases pain
- Prevents heart disease
- Lowers stress hormones
- Relaxes your muscles

Mental Health Benefits

- Adds joy and zest to life
- Relieves stress
- Enhances resilience
- Eases anxiety and fear
- Improves mood

Social Benefits

- Strengthens relationships
- Enhances teamwork
- Promotes group bonding
- Attracts others to us
- Helps defuse conflict

Laughter And Humor Help You Stay Emotionally Healthy

Laughter makes you feel good. And the good feeling that you get when you laugh remains with you even after the laughter subsides. Humor helps you keep a positive, optimistic outlook through difficult situations, disappointments, and loss.

More than just a respite from sadness and pain, laughter gives you the courage and strength to find new sources of meaning and hope. Even in the most difficult of times, a laugh—or even simply a smile—can go a long way toward making you feel better. And laughter really is contagious—just hearing laughter primes your brain and readies you to smile and join in the fun.

The Link Between Laughter And Mental Health

- **Laughter dissolves distressing emotions.** You can't feel anxious, angry, or sad when you're laughing.

- **Laughter helps you relax and recharge.** It reduces stress and increases energy, enabling you to stay focused and accomplish more.

- **Humor shifts perspective.** [It allows] you to see situations in a more realistic, less threatening light. A humorous perspective creates psychological distance, which can help you avoid feeling overwhelmed.

The Social Benefits Of Humor And Laughter

Humor and playful communication strengthen our relationships by triggering positive feelings and fostering emotional connection. When we laugh with one another, a positive bond is created. This bond acts as a strong buffer against stress, disagreements, and disappointment.

Laughing With Others Is More Powerful Than Laughing Alone

Shared laughter is one of the most effective tools for keeping relationships fresh and exciting. All emotional sharing builds strong and lasting relationship bonds, but sharing laughter and play also adds joy, vitality, and resilience. And humor is a powerful and effective way to heal resentments, disagreements, and hurts. Laughter unites people during difficult times.

Incorporating more humor and play into your daily interactions can improve the quality of your love relationships—as well as your connections with co-workers, family members, and friends. Using humor and laughter in relationships allows you to:

- **Be more spontaneous** (Humor gets you out of your head and away from your troubles.);

- **Let go of defensiveness** (Laughter helps you forget judgments, criticisms, and doubts);

- **Release inhibitions** (Your fear of holding back and holding on are set aside); and

- **Express your true feelings** (Deeply felt emotions are allowed to rise to the surface.).

Bringing More Humor And Laughter Into Your Life

Laughter is your birthright, a natural part of life that is innate and inborn. Infants begin smiling during the first weeks of life and laugh out loud within months of being born. Even if you did not grow up in a household where laughter was a common sound, you can learn to laugh at any stage of life.

Begin by setting aside special times to seek out humor and laughter, as you might with working out, and build from there. Eventually, you'll want to incorporate humor and laughter into the fabric of your life, finding it naturally in everything you do.

Here are some ways to start:

- **Smile.** Smiling is the beginning of laughter. Like laughter, it's contagious. Pioneers in "laugh therapy," find it's possible to laugh without even experiencing a funny event. The

Creating Opportunities To Laugh

- Watch a funny movie or TV show.
- Go to a comedy club.
- Read the funny pages.
- Seek out funny people.
- Share a good joke or a funny story.
- Check out your bookstore's humor section.
- Host game night with friends.
- Play with a pet.
- Go to a "laughter yoga" class.
- Goof around with children.
- Do something silly.
- Make time for fun activities (e.g., bowling, miniature golfing, karaoke).

Want To Bring The Fun? Get A Pet...

Most of us have experienced the joy of playing with a furry friend, and pets are a rewarding way to bring more laughter and joy into your life. But did you know that having a pet is also good for your mental and physical health? Studies show that pets can protect you depression, stress, and even heart disease.

same holds for smiling. When you look at someone or see something even mildly pleasing, practice smiling.

- **Count your blessings.** Literally make a list. The simple act of considering the good things in your life will distance you from negative thoughts that are a barrier to humor and laughter. When you're in a state of sadness, you have further to travel to get to humor and laughter.

- **When you hear laughter, move toward it.** Sometimes humor and laughter are private, a shared joke among a small group, but usually not. More often, people are very happy to share something funny because it gives them an opportunity to laugh again and feed off the humor you find in it. When you hear laughter, seek it out and ask, "What's funny?"

- **Spend time with fun, playful people.** These are people who laugh easily—both at themselves and at life's absurdities—and who routinely find the humor in everyday events. Their playful point of view and laughter are contagious.

- **Bring humor into conversations.** Ask people, "What's the funniest thing that happened to you today? This week? In your life?"

Developing Your Sense Of Humor: Take Yourself Less Seriously

One essential characteristic that helps us laugh is not taking ourselves too seriously. We've all known the classic tight-jawed sourpuss who takes everything with deathly seriousness and never laughs at anything. No fun there!

Some events are clearly sad and not occasions for laughter. But most events in life don't carry an overwhelming sense of either sadness or delight. They fall into the gray zone of ordinary life—giving you the choice to laugh or not.

Ways To Help Yourself See The Lighter Side Of Life

- **Laugh at yourself.** Share your embarrassing moments. The best way to take yourself less seriously is to talk about times when you took yourself too seriously.

- **Attempt to laugh at situations rather than bemoan them.** Look for the humor in a bad situation, and uncover the irony and absurdity of life. This will help improve your mood and the mood of those around you.

- **Surround yourself with reminders to lighten up.** Keep a toy on your desk or in your car. Put up a funny poster in your office. Choose a computer screensaver that makes you laugh. Frame photos of you and your family or friends having fun.

- **Keep things in perspective.** Many things in life are beyond your control—particularly the behavior of other people. While you might think taking the weight of the world on your shoulders is admirable, in the long run it's unrealistic, unproductive, unhealthy, and even egotistical.

- **Deal with your stress.** Stress is a major impediment to humor and laughter.

- **Pay attention to children and emulate them.** They are the experts on playing, taking life lightly, and laughing.

Checklist For Lightening Up

When you find yourself taken over by what seems to be a horrible problem, ask these questions:

- Is it really worth getting upset over?
- Is it worth upsetting others?
- Is it that important?
- Is it that bad?
- Is the situation irreparable?
- Is it really your problem?

Using Humor And Play To Overcome Challenges And Enhance Your Life

The ability to laugh, play, and have fun with others not only makes life more enjoyable but also helps you solve problems, connect with others, and be more creative. People who incorporate humor and play into their daily lives find that it renews them and all of their relationships.

Life brings challenges that can either get the best of you or become playthings for your imagination. When you "become the problem" and take yourself too seriously, it can be hard to think outside the box and find new solutions. But when you play with the problem, you can often transform it into an opportunity for creative learning.

Playing with problems seems to come naturally to children. When they are confused or afraid, they make their problems into a game, giving them a sense of control and an opportunity to experiment with new solutions. Interacting with others in playful ways helps you retain this creative ability.

Here are two examples of people who took everyday problems and turned them around through laughter and play:

- Roy, a semi-retired businessman, was excited to finally have time to devote to golf, his favorite sport. But the more he played, the less he enjoyed himself. Although his game had improved dramatically, he got angry with himself over every mistake. Roy wisely realized that his golfing buddies affected his attitude, so he stopped playing with people who took the game too seriously. When he played with friends who focused more on having fun than on their scores, he was less critical of himself. Now golfing was as enjoyable as Roy hoped it would be. He scored better without working harder. And the brighter outlook he was getting from his companions and the game spread to other parts of his life, including his work.

- Jane worked at home designing greeting cards, a job she used to love but now felt had become routine. Two little girls who loved to draw and paint lived next door. Eventually, Jane invited the girls in to play with all the art supplies she had. At first, she just watched, but in time she joined in. Laughing, coloring, and playing pretend with the little girls transformed Jane's life. Not only did playing with them end her loneliness and mild boredom, it sparked her imagination and helped her artwork flourish. Best of all, it rekindled the playfulness and spark in Jane's relationship with her husband.

As laughter, humor, and play become an integrated part of your life, your creativity will flourish and new discoveries for playing with friends, coworkers, acquaintances, and loved ones will occur to you daily. Humor takes you to a higher place where you can view the world from a more relaxed, positive, creative, joyful, and balanced perspective.

Chapter 58

Interacting With Pets

When thinking of ways to reduce stress in life, usually techniques like meditation, yoga and journaling come to mind. These are great techniques, to be sure. But getting a new best friend can also have many stress relieving and health benefits. While human friends provide great social support and come with some fabulous benefits, this article focuses on the benefits of furry friends: cats and dogs!

Research shows that, unless you're someone who really dislikes animals or is absolutely too busy to care for one properly, pets can provide excellent social support, stress relief and other health benefits—perhaps more than people! Here are more health benefits of pets:

Pets Can Improve Your Mood

For those who love animals, it's virtually impossible to stay in a bad mood when a pair of loving puppy eyes meets yours, or when a super-soft cat rubs up against your hand. Research supports the mood-enhancing benefits of pets. A recent study found that men with AIDS were less likely to suffer from depression if they owned a pet. (According to one study, men with AIDS who did not own a pet were about three times more likely to report symptoms of depression than men who did not have AIDS. But men with AIDS who had pets were only about 50 percent more likely to report symptoms of depression, as compared to men in the study who did not have AIDS.)

About This Chapter: "How Owning a Dog or Cat Can Reduce Stress," http://stress.about.com/od/lowstresslifestyle/a/petsandstress.htm. © 2013 Elizabeth Scott, M.S. (http://stress.about.com/). Used with permission of About Inc., which can be found online at www.about.com. All rights reserved.

Pets Control Blood Pressure Better Than Drugs

Yes, it's true. While [angiotensin-converting-enzyme] ACE inhibiting drugs can generally reduce blood pressure, they aren't as effective on controlling spikes in blood pressure due to stress and tension. However, in a recent study, groups of hypertensive New York stockbrokers who got dogs or cats were found to have lower blood pressure and heart rates than those who didn't get pets. When they heard of the results, most of those in the non-pet group went out and got pets!

Pets Encourage You To Get Out And Exercise

Whether we walk our dogs because they need it, or are more likely to enjoy a walk when we have companionship, dog owners do spend more time walking than non-pet owners, at least if we live in an urban setting. Because exercise is good for stress management and overall health, owning ado can be credited with increasing these benefits.

Pets Can Help With Social Support

When we're out walking, having a dog with us can make us more approachable and give people a reason to stop and talk, thereby increasing the number of people we meet, giving us an opportunity to increase our network of friends and acquaintances, which also has great stress management benefits.

Pets Stave Off Loneliness And Provide Unconditional Love

Pets can be there for you in ways that people can't. They can offer love and companionship, and can also enjoy comfortable silences, keep secrets, and are excellent snugglers. And they could be the best antidote to loneliness. In fact, research shows that nursing home residents reported less loneliness when visited by dogs than when they spent time with other people! All these benefits can reduce the amount of stress people experience in response to feelings of social isolation and lack of social support from people.

Pets Can Reduce Stress—Sometimes More Than People

While we all know the power of talking about your problems with a good friend who's also a good listener, recent research shows that spending time with a pet may be even better! Recent research shows that, when conducting a task that's stressful, people actually experienced less stress when their pets were with them than when a supportive friend or even their spouse was present! (This may be partially due to the fact that pets don't judge us; they just love us.)

It's important to realize that owning a pet isn't for everyone. Pets do come with additional work and responsibility, which can bring its own stress.

However, for most people, the benefits of having a pet outweigh the drawbacks. Having a furry best friend can reduce stress in your life and bring you support when times get tough.

Chapter 59

Art Therapies

For thousands of years, people have searched for the meaning and beauty of life in music, painting, poetry, and other arts. Now scientists are finding that the arts can benefit both your mental and physical health.

Current research is following a number of paths. Some scientists measure the natural substances your body produces when you're listening to music or otherwise exposed to the arts. Others look at what happens when you are active in the creative process. Researchers are now investigating how the arts can help us recover from disease, injury and psychological trauma. Many scientists agree that the arts can help reduce stress and anxiety, improve well-being and enhance the way we fight infection.

Music Therapy

Let's start with music. "There is a reward system in place for learning music," says Dr. Daniel Levitin of McGill University in Montréal. Music can activate the same brain areas as chocolate and opium—of course, at different intensities.

Music plays an important role throughout our lives. Parents worldwide sing and coo to their babies. And let's not forget the other end of the life cycle: Levitin says that music "may be the last thing to go" in those with severe memory loss from Alzheimer's disease. "Even if they don't know their own spouse, they can sing the songs of their youth."

About This Chapter: The information in this chapter is excerpted from "More Than A Feeling: How The Arts Affect Your Health," *News In Health* (www.newsinhealth.nih.gov), National Institutes of Health, June 2008. Reviewed by David A. Cooke, MD, FACP, April 2013.

Recent studies have found evidence that singing releases substances that serve as the brain's own natural painkillers. Singing also increases the "bonding hormone" that helps us feel a sense of trust. And when we listen to music, levels of molecules important for fighting infection can rise.

Many of us intuitively use music for relaxation and enjoyment—to socialize, exercise, or change our mood after a hard day. But music therapy is sometimes used in the clinic, as well, requiring a certified therapist to interact with the patient.

To measure the effects of such therapy, one study showed how levels of an important brain chemical that relays signals between cells increased after four weeks of music therapy. It then decreased after the therapy was halted.

And a recent report from Finnish scientists showed that listening to music helps stroke patients recover both memory and focused attention. The researchers also found that music can reduce post-stroke depression and confusion. Other studies suggest that stroke patients may improve faster if they sing, rather than speak, as part of their rehabilitation.

Art Therapy

Scientists are also studying how art therapy can help to ease pain and stress and improve quality of life. Megan Robb, a certified art therapist at the National Institutes of Health (NIH)'s Clinical Center, says, "When traumatic memories are stored in the brain, they're not stored as words but as images. Art therapy is uniquely suited to access these memories."

Once you draw or paint these images, she explains, you can then progress to forming words to describe them. This externalizes the trauma—moves it out of isolation, onto the page and into a positive exchange with the therapist. This process, Robb says, gives you "an active involvement in your own healing."

Several small studies, some of which were supported by the National Institutes of Health (NIH), have suggested that art therapy can help improve health status, quality of life, and coping behaviors. It can improve depression and fatigue in cancer patients on chemotherapy, and help prevent burnout in caregivers. It's also been used to help prepare children for painful medical procedures, as well as to improve the speech of children with cerebral palsy.

Writing Therapy

And then there's writing. Expressive writing—writing about traumatic, stressful or emotional events—has been shown to have a number of health benefits, from improving symptoms of depression to helping fight infection. Dr. James W. Pennebaker of the University of Texas at Austin has designed several studies to show the links between writing and health.

"Writing about emotional upheavals in our lives can improve physical and mental health," Pennebaker says. "Although the scientific research surrounding the value of expressive writing is still in the early phases, there are some approaches to writing that have been found to be helpful."

In a series of exercises, healthy student volunteers who wrote about traumatic experiences had more positive moods, fewer illnesses and better measures of immune-system function than those who wrote about superficial experiences. Even six weeks later, the students who'd written about what upset them reported more positive moods and fewer illnesses than those who'd written about everyday experiences.

In another study of students vulnerable to depression, those who did expressive writing exercises showed significantly lower depression symptoms, even after six months, than those who had written about everyday matters.

Movement Therapy

Arts that involve movement, such as dance, can also bring health benefits. Researchers already know that physical activity can help you reduce stress, gain energy, sleep better, and fight

---

Wise Choices: Arts For Health

The arts may bring more than intellectual benefits. Recent research suggests they may help your physical and mental health.

Try these for a start:

- Write for at least 15 minutes a day, for at least three consecutive days, about something that worries or bothers you. If it makes you feel too upset, simply stop writing or change topics. Experiment to find what works best for you.

- Listen to music to reduce stress and improve quality of life.

- Try a dance class or Tai Chi, a sequence of slow, graceful body movements. These kinds of movements can help reduce stress.

- Try doodling or drawing as a way to work out tension.

depression and anxiety. NIH-funded researchers are now studying tai chi—a sequence of slow, graceful body movements—to see how it affects fitness and stress in cancer survivors.

Studies

NIH is currently funding several studies to learn more about the health effects of expressive writing and other arts. If you're interested in participating, search for clinical trials in your area at http://clinicaltrials.gov.

Remember that the arts are no substitute for medical help when you need it. But they can still bring health benefits. If you enjoy writing or any other art, go for it. You don't have to be "good" at them for them to be good for you.

Chapter 60

Health Benefits Of Journaling

I'll bet you write (or word process) daily. If you are like most women, you record only what you must. In an effort to change your mind and your habits, I'll let you in on a well-kept secret: A pen coupled with paper can serve as a powerful life tool.

Journaling (or keeping letters or diaries) is an ancient tradition, one that dates back to at least 10th century Japan. Successful people throughout history have kept journals. Presidents have maintained them for posterity; other famous figures for their own purposes. Oscar Wilde, 19th century playwright, said: "I never travel without my diary. One should always have something sensational to read on the train."

Health Benefits

Contrary to popular belief, our forefathers (and mothers) did know a thing or two. There is increasing evidence to support the notion that journaling has a positive impact on physical well-being. University of Texas at Austin psychologist and researcher James Pennebaker contends that regular journaling strengthens immune cells, called T-lymphocytes. Other research indicates that journaling decreases the symptoms of asthma and rheumatoid arthritis. Pennebaker believes that writing about stressful events helps you come to terms with them, thus reducing the impact of these stressors on your physical health.

About This Chapter: Information for this chapter is reprinted from "The Health Benefits of Journaling," by Maud Purcell, LCSW, CEAP. © 2013 PsychCentral (www.psychcentral.com). All rights reserved. Reprinted with permission.

I know what you're thinking: "So writing a few sentences a day may keep me healthier longer, but so will eating lima beans! Why should I bother journaling when I've already got too much on my plate?" The following facts may convince you.

Scientific evidence supports that journaling provides other unexpected benefits. The act of writing accesses your left brain, which is analytical and rational. While your left brain is occupied, your right brain is free to create, intuit, and feel. In sum, writing removes mental blocks and allows you to use all of your brainpower to better understand yourself, others, and the world around you. Begin journaling and begin experiencing these benefits:

Blogging May Help Teens Dealing With Social Distress

Teens blogging about social problems, engaging with online community showed significant improvement, according to new research.

Blogging may have psychological benefits for teens suffering from social anxiety, improving their self-esteem and helping them relate better to their friends, according to new research published by the American Psychological Association.

"Research has shown that writing a personal diary and other forms of expressive writing are a great way to release emotional distress and just feel better," said the study's lead author, Meyran Boniel-Nissim, PhD, of the University of Haifa, Israel. "Teens are online anyway, so blogging enables free expression and easy communication with others."

Maintaining a blog had a stronger positive effect on troubled students' well-being than merely expressing their social anxieties and concerns in a private diary, according to the article published online in the APA journal *Psychological Services*. Opening the blog up to comments from the online community intensified those effects.

"Although cyberbullying and online abuse are extensive and broad, we noted that almost all responses to our participants' blog messages were supportive and positive in nature," said the study's co-author, Azy Barak, PhD. "We weren't surprised, as we frequently see positive social expressions online in terms of generosity, support, and advice."

The researchers randomly surveyed high school students in Israel, who had agreed to fill out a questionnaire about their feelings on the quality of their social relationships. A total of 161 students—124 girls and 37 boys, with an average age of 15—were selected because their scores on the survey showed they all had some level of social anxiety or distress. All the teens reported difficulty making friends or relating to the friends they had. The researchers assessed the teens' self-esteem, everyday social activities, and behaviors before, immediately after, and two months after the 10-week experiment.

- **Clarify your thoughts and feelings.** Do you ever seem all jumbled up inside, unsure of what you want or feel? Taking a few minutes to jot down your thoughts and emotions (no editing!) will quickly get you in touch with your internal world.

- **Know yourself better.** By writing routinely you will get to know what makes you feel happy and confident. You will also become clear about situations and people who are toxic for you—important information for your emotional well-being.

- **Reduce stress.** Writing about anger, sadness, and other painful emotions helps to release the intensity of these feelings. By doing so, you will feel calmer and better able to stay in the present.

Four groups of students were assigned to blog. Two of those groups were told to focus their posts on their social problems, with one group opening the posts to comments; the other two groups could write about whatever they wanted and, again, one group opened the blog up to comments. The number and content of comments were not evaluated for this experiment. The students could respond to comments but that was not required. Two more groups acted as controls—either writing a private diary about their social problems or doing nothing. Participants in the writing and blogging groups were told to post messages at least twice a week for 10 weeks.

Four experts, who held masters or doctoral degrees in counseling and psychology, assessed the bloggers' social and emotional condition via their blog posts. Students were assessed as having a poor social and emotional state if they wrote extensively about personal problems or bad relationships or showed evidence of low self-esteem, for example.

Self-esteem, social anxiety, emotional distress, and the number of positive social behaviors improved significantly for the bloggers when compared to the teens who did nothing and those who wrote private diaries. Bloggers who were instructed to write specifically about their difficulties and whose blogs were open to comments improved the most. All of these results were consistent at the two month follow-up.

The authors conceded that the skewed sex ratio was a limitation to the study. However, the researchers analyzed the results separately by gender and found that boys and girls reacted similarly to the interventions and there were no major differences. However, they say future research should attempt to control for gender.

- **Solve problems more effectively.** Typically we problem solve from a left-brained, analytical perspective. But sometimes the answer can only be found by engaging right-brained creativity and intuition. Writing unlocks these other capabilities, and affords the opportunity for unexpected solutions to seemingly unsolvable problems.

- **Resolve disagreements with others.** Writing about misunderstandings rather than stewing over them will help you to understand another's point of view. And you just may come up with a sensible resolution to the conflict.

In addition to all of these wonderful benefits, keeping a journal allows you to track patterns, trends, and improvement and growth over time. When current circumstances appear insurmountable, you will be able to look back on previous dilemmas that you have since resolved.

How To Begin

Your journaling will be most effective if you do it daily for about 20 minutes. Begin anywhere, and forget spelling and punctuation. Privacy is key if you are to write without censor. Write quickly, as this frees your brain from "should" and other blocks to successful journaling. If it helps, pick a theme for the day, week, or month (for example, peace of mind, confusion, change, or anger). The most important rule of all is that there are no rules.

Through your writing, you'll discover that your journal is an all-accepting, nonjudgmental friend. And she may provide the cheapest therapy you will ever get. Best of luck on your journaling journey!

Part Six
If You Need More Information

Chapter 61

Directory Of Stress And Stress Management Resources

American Academy of Allergy, Asthma, and Immunology

555 East Wells Street, Suite 1100
Milwaukee, WI 53202-3823
Phone: 414-272-6071
Website: www.aaaai.org
E-mail: info@aaaai.org

American Academy of Child and Adolescent Psychiatry

3615 Wisconsin Avenue NW
Washington, DC 20016-3007
Phone: 202-966-7300
Fax: 202-966-2891
Website: www.aacap.org
E-mail: communications@aacap.org

American Academy of Dermatology

P.O. Box 4014
Schaumburg, IL 60618-4014
Toll-Free: 866-503-SKIN (866-503-7546)
Phone: 847-240-1280
Fax: 847-240-1859
Website: www.aad.org
E-mail: MRC@aad.org

American Academy of Experts in Traumatic Stress

203 Deer Road
Ronkonkoma, NY 11779
Phone: 631-543-2217
Fax: 631-543-6977
Website: www.aaets.org
E-mail: info@aaets.org

About This Chapter: Information in this chapter was compiled from many sources deemed reliable; inclusion does not constitute endorsement. All contact information was verified and updated in April 2013.

American Academy of Family Physicians

P.O. Box 11210
Shawnee Mission, KS 66207-1210
Toll-Free: 800-274-2237
Phone: 913-906-6000
Fax: 913-906-6075
Website: www.aafp.org
E-mail: contactcenter@aafp.org

American Heart Association

7272 Greenville Avenue
Dallas, TX 75231
Toll-Free: 800-AHA-USA-1
(800-242-8721)
Phone: 214-373-6300
Website: www.americanheart.org
E-mail: inquiries@heart.org

American Institute of Stress

9112 Camp Bowie West Blvd., #228
Fort Worth, TX 76116
Phone: 682-239-6823
Fax: 817-394-0593
Website: www.stress.org
E-mail: info@stress.org

American Massage Therapy Association

500 Davis Street, Suite 900
Evanston, IL 60201-4695
Toll-Free: 877-905-0577
Phone: 847-864-0123
Fax: 847-864-5196
Website: www.amtamassage.org
E-mail: info@amtamassage.org

American Meditation Institute

60 Garner Road, P.O. Box 430
Averill Park, NY 12018
Toll-Free: 800-234-5115
Phone/Fax: 518-674-8714
Website: www.americanmeditation.org
E-mail: ami@americanmeditation.org

American Psychiatric Association

1000 Wilson Boulevard, Suite 1825
Arlington, VA 22209-3901
Toll-Free: 888-35-PSYCH
(888-357-7924)
Phone: 703-907-7300
Website: www.psych.org
E-mail: apa@psych.org

American Psychological Association (APA)

750 First Street NE
Washington, DC 20002-4242
Toll-Free: 800-374-2721
Phone: 202-336-5500
TDD/TTY: 202-336-6123
Website: www.apa.org
E-mail: public.affairs@apa.org

American Foundation for Suicide Prevention

120 Wall Street, 29th Floor
New York, NY 10005
Toll-Free: 888-333-AFSP (2377)
Phone: 212-363-3500
Fax: 212-363-6237
Website: www.afsp.org
E-mail: info@afsp.org

American Yoga Association

P.O. Box 19986
Sarasota, FL 34276
Fax: 941-921-4977
Website: www.americanyogaassociation.org
E-mail: info@americanyogaassociation.org

Anxiety and Depression Association of America

8701 Georgia Avenue, Suite 412
Silver Spring, MD 20910
Phone: 240-485-1001
Fax: 240-485-1035
Website: www.adaa.org
E-mail: information@adaa.org

Association for Behavioral and Cognitive Therapies

305 7th Avenue, 16th Floor
New York, NY 10001
Phone: 212-647-1890
Fax: 212-647-1865
Website: https://www.abct.org

Better Health Channel

GPO Box 4057, Melbourne 3001
Victoria 3000
Australia
Website: www.betterhealth.vic.gov.au

Center for Young Women's Health

333 Longwood Avenue, 5th floor
Boston, MA 02115 USA
Phone: 617-355-2994
Fax: 617-730-0186
Website: www.youngwomenshealth.org

Centers for Disease Control and Prevention (CDC)

1600 Clifton Road
Atlanta, GA 30333
Toll-Free: 800-CDC-INFO
(800-232-4636)
Toll-Free TTY: 888-232-6348
Phone: 404-639-3534
Website: www.cdc.gov

Cleveland Clinic

9500 Euclid Avenue
Cleveland, OH 44195
Toll-Free: 800-223-CARE
(800-223-2273)
TTY: 216-444-0261
Website: www.clevelandclinic.org

Cool Spot

National Institute on
Alcohol Abuse and Alcoholism
5635 Fishers Lane
Room 3098
MSC 9304
Bethesda, MD 20892-9304
Website: www.thecoolspot.gov
E-mail: niaaaweb-r@exchange.nih.gov

CopeCareDeal

Website: www.copecaredeal.org

FamilyDoctor.org

Website: www.familydoctor.org

GirlsHealth.gov

U.S. Department of Health
and Human Services
200 Independence Avenue SW
Room 712E
Washington, DC 20201
Website: www.girlshealth.gov

HealthFinder.gov

National Health Information Center
P.O. Box 1133
Washington, DC 20013-1133
Toll-Free: 800-336-4797
Phone: 240-453-8280
Website: healthfinder.gov
E-mail:
healthfinder@nhic.org or info@nhic.org

HealthyChildren.org

American Academy of Pediatrics
141 Northwest Point Boulevard
Elk Grove Village, IL 60007-1098
Phone: 847-434-4000
Fax: 847-434-8000
Website: Healthychildren.org
E-mail: info@healthychildren.org

International Society for Traumatic Stress Studies

111 Deer Lake Road, Suite 100
Deerfield, IL 60015
Phone: 847-480-9028
Fax: 847-480-9282
Website: www.istss.org
E-mail: istss@istss.org

It's My Life

Website: pbskids.org/itsmylife
E-mail: itsmylife@pbs.org

Maternal and Family Health Services

15 Public Square
Suite 600
Wilkes-Barre, PA 18701
Toll-Free: 800-367-6347
Phone: 570-826-1777
Fax: 570-823-3040
Website: www.mfhs.org
E-mail: info@mfhs.org

Mental Health America

2000 North Beauregard Street
6th Floor
Alexandria, VA 22311
Toll-Free: 800-969-6642
Toll-Free TTY: 800-433-5959
Phone: 703-684-7722
Fax: 703-684-5968
Website:
www.mentalhealthamerica.net
E-mail:
info@mentalhealthamerica.net

National Alliance on Mental Illness (NAMI)

3803 North Fairfax Drive
Suite 100
Arlington, VA 22203
Toll-Free: 800-950-NAMI
(800-950-6264—Information Helpline)
Phone: 703-524-7600
Fax: 703-524-9094
Website: www.nami.org
E-mail: info@nami.org

National Cancer Institute (NCI)

NCI Public Inquiries Office
6116 Executive Boulevard
Suite 300
Bethesda, MD 20892-8322
Toll-Free: 800-4-CANCER
(800-422-6237)
Toll-Free TTY: 800-332-8615
Website: www.cancer.gov
E-mail: cancergovstaff@mail.nih.gov

National Center for Complementary and Alternative Medicine (NCCAM)

9000 Rockville Pike
Bethesda, MD 20892
Toll-Free: 888-644-6226
Toll-Free TTY: 866-464-3615
Toll-Free Fax: 866-464-3616
Website: nccam.nih.gov
E-mail: info@nccam.nih.gov

National Eczema Society

Hill House
Highgate Hill
London
N19 5NA
Website: www.eczema.org
E-mail: helpline@eczema.org

National Institute on Alcohol Abuse and Alcoholism (NIAAA)

National Institutes of Health
5635 Fishers Lane, MSC 9304
Bethesda, MD 20892-9304
Toll-Free: 888-MY-NIAAA
(888-696-4222)
Website: www.niaaa.nih.gov
Website: pubs.niaaa.nih.gov/publications/
english-order.htm (for NIAAA publications)
E-mail: niaaaweb-r@exchange.nih.gov

National Institute of Allergy and Infectious Diseases

Office of Communications
and Public Liaison
6610 Rockledge Drive, MSC 6612
Bethesda, MD 20892-6612
Toll-Free: 866-284-4107
Toll-Free TDD: 800-877-8339
Phone: 301-496-5717
Fax: 301-402-3573
Website: www.niaid.nih.gov
E-mail:
ocpostoffice@niaid.nih.gov

369

National Institute of Arthritis and Musculoskeletal and Skin Diseases (NIAMS)

Information Clearinghouse
National Institutes of Health
1 AMS Circle
Bethesda, MD 20892-3675
Toll-Free: 877-22-NIAMS
(877-226-4267)
Phone: 301-495-4484
TTY: 301-565-2966
Fax: 301-718-6366
Website: www.niams.nih.gov
E-mail: NIAMSinfo@mail.nih.gov

National Institute of Child Health and Human Development (NICHD)

31 Center Drive
Building 31, Room 2A32
Bethesda, MD 20892-2425
Toll-Free: 800-370-2943
Toll-Free TTY: 888-320-6942
Toll-Free Fax: 866-760-5947
Fax: 301-984-1473
Website: www.nichd.nih.gov
E-mail: NICHDInformation
ResourceCenter@mail.nih.gov

National Institute of Diabetes and Digestive and Kidney Diseases (NIDDK)

Office of Communications
and Public Liaison
Building 31, Room 9A06
31 Center Drive, MSC 2560
Bethesda, MD 20892-2560
Phone: 301-496-3583
Website: www2.niddk.nih.gov

National Institute on Drug Abuse (NIDA)

Office of Science Policy and Communications, Public Information and Liaison Branch
6001 Executive Boulevard
Room 5213, MSC 9561
Bethesda, MD 20892-9561
Phone: 301-443-1124
Website: www.drugabuse.gov

National Institutes of Health (NIH)

9000 Rockville Pike
Bethesda, MD 20892
Phone: 301-496-4000
TTY: 301-402-9612
Website: www.nih.gov
E-mail: NIHinfo@od.nih.gov

National Institute of General Medical Sciences (NIGMS)

45 Center Drive, MSC 6200
Bethesda, MD 20892-6200
Phone: 301-496-7301
Website: www.nigms.nih.gov
E-mail: info@nigms.nih.gov

National Institute of Mental Health (NIMH)

Science Writing, Press,
and Dissemination Branch
6001 Executive Boulevard
Room 8184, MSC 9663
Bethesda, MD 20892-9663
Toll-Free: 866-615-NIMH
(866-615-6464)
Toll-Free TTY: 866-415-8051
Phone: 301-443-4513
TTY: 301-443-8431
Fax: 301-443-4279
Website: www.nimh.nih.gov
E-mail: nimhinfo@nih.gov

National Library of Medicine (NLM)

8600 Rockville Pike
Bethesda, MD 20894
Toll-Free: 888-FIND-NLM
(888-346-3656)
Toll-Free TDD: 800-735-2258
(TDD access via
Maryland Relay Service)
Phone: 301-594-5983
Fax: 301-402-1384
Website: www.nlm.nih.gov

National Multiple Sclerosis Society

733 Third Avenue, 3rd Floor
New York, NY 10017
Toll-Free: 800-344-4867
Website:
www.nationalmssociety.org

National Institute of Neurological Disorders and Stroke

NIH Neurological Institute
P.O. Box 5801
Bethesda, MD 20824
Toll-Free: 800-352-9424
Phone: 301-496-5751
Website: www.ninds.nih.gov

National Science Foundation

4201 Wilson Boulevard
Arlington, VA 22230
Toll-Free TDD: 800-281-8749
Phone: 703-292-5111
TDD: 703-292-5090
Website: www.nsf.gov
E-mail: info@nsf.gov

National Sleep Foundation

1010 North Glebe Road, Suite 310
Arlington, VA 22201
Phone: 703-243-1697
Website: www.sleepfoundation.org
E-mail: nsf@sleepfoundation.org

National Women's Health Information Center

Department of Health
and Human Services
200 Independence Avenue SW, Room 712E
Washington, DC 20201
Toll-Free: 800-994-9662
Toll-Free TDD: 888-220-5446
Phone: 202-690-7650
Fax: 202-205-2631
Website: www.womenshealth.gov
E-mail: womenshealth@hhs.gov

Nemours Foundation

1600 Rockland Road
Wilmington, DE 19803
Phone: 302-651-4000
Website: www.kidshealth.org
E-mail: info@kidshealth.org

North American Spine Society

7075 Veterans Boulevard
Burr Ridge, IL 60527
Toll-Free: 866-960-6277
Phone: 630-230-3600
Fax: 630-230-3700
Website: www.knowyourback.org

Office on Women's Health

Department of Health
and Human Services
200 Independence Avenue SW
Room 712E
Washington, DC 20201
Toll-Free: 800-994-9662
Phone: 202-690-7650
Fax: 202-205-2631
Website: www.womenshealth.gov

Palo Alto Medical Foundation

2025 Soquel Avenue
Santa Cruz, CA 95062
Toll-Free: 888-398-5677
Phone: 831-423-4111
Website: www.pamf.org
E-mail: communityrelations@pamf.org

Phoenix House

Toll-Free: 888-286-5027
Website: www.phoenixhouse.org

PsychCentral

55 Pleasant Street, Suite 207
Newburyport, MA 01950
Website: psychcentral.com
E-mail: talkback@psychcentral.com

Ready Campaign

FEMA/DHS
500 C Street SW
Suite 714
Washington, DC 20472
Toll-Free: 800-621-FEMA
(800-621-3362)
Toll-Free TTY: 800-462-7585
Website: www.ready.gov/kids
E-mail: ready@fema.gov

S.A.F.E. ALTERNATIVES

Toll-Free: 800-DONTCUT
(800-366-8288)
Toll-Free Fax: 888-296-7988
Website: www.selfinjury.com
E-mail: info@selfinjury.com

Safe Teens

Toll-Free: 866-SAFETEENS
(866-723-3833)
Website: www.safeteens.org
E-mail: info@safeteens.org

SAMHSA's Health Information Network

P.O. Box 2345
Rockville, MD 20847-2345
Toll-Free: 877-SAMHSA-7
(877-726-4727)
Toll-Free TTY: 800-487-4889
Fax: 240-221-4292
Website: store.samhsa.gov
E-mail: SAMHSAInfo@samhsa.hhs.gov

StopBullying.gov

U.S. Department of Health
and Human Services
200 Independence Avenue SW
Washington, DC 20201
Website: www.stopbullying.gov

Students Against Destructive Decisions (SADD)

255 Main Street
Marlborough, MA 01752
Toll-Free: 877-SADD-INC
(877-723-3462)
Fax: 508-481-5759
Website: www.sadd.org
E-mail: info@sadd.org

United Advocates for Children and Families

2035 Hurley Way
Suite 290
Sacramento, CA 95825
Toll-Free: 866-643-1530 or
877-ASK UACF (877-275-8223)
Phone: 916-643-1530
Fax: 916-643-1592
Website: www.uacf4hope.org
E-mail: info@uacf4hope.org

U.S. Department of Health and Human Services (HHS)

200 Independence Avenue SW
Washington, DC 20201
Toll-Free: 877-696-6775
Website: www.hhs.gov

U.S. Department of Veterans Affairs

810 Vermont Avenue NW
Washington, DC 20420
Toll-Free: 800-827-1000
Toll-Free TDD: 800-829-4833
Website: www.va.gov

Women's and Children's Health Network

295 South Terrace, Adelaide
South Australia 5000
Website: www.cyh.com

Young Men's Health

333 Longwood Avenue, 5th floor
Boston, MA 02115
Website: www.youngmenshealthsite.org
E-mail: ymh@childrens.harvard.edu

Chapter 62

Additional Reading About Stress And Stress Management

Books

A Teen's Guide to Success: How to Be Calm, Confident, Focused
By Ben Bernstein, PhD; Published by Familius, 2013; ISBN: 978-1938301186

Balancing Act: A Teen's Guide to Managing Stress
By Joan Esherick; Published by Mason Crest Publishers, 2005;
ISBN: 978-1590848531

Dealing With Stress: A How-To Guide
By Lisa A. Wroble; Published by Enslow Publisher, 2011; ISBN: 978-1598453096

Dealing With the Stuff That Makes Life Tough:
The 10 Things That Stress Girls Out and How to Cope with Them
By Jill Zimmerman Rutledge; Published by McGraw-Hill, 2004; ISBN: 978-0071423267

Don't Sweat the Small Stuff for Teens:
Simple Ways to Keep Your Cool in Stressful Times
By Richard Carlson, PhD; Published by Hyperion, 2000;
ISBN: 978-0786885978

About This Chapter: This chapter includes a compilation of various resources from many sources deemed reliable. It serves as a starting point for further research and is not intended to be comprehensive. Inclusion does not constitute endorsement. Resources in this chapter are categorized by type and, under each type, they are listed alphabetically by title to make topics easier to identify. List compiled in April 2013.

Don't Worry, You'll Get In:
100 Winning Tips for Stress-Free College Admissions

By Mimi Doe and Michele A. Hernandez; Published by Marlowe and Company, 2005; ISBN: 978-1569243671

The Drama Years: Real Girls Talk About Surviving Middle School—Bullies, Brands, Body Image, and More

By Haley Kilpatrick and Whitney Joiner; Published by Free Press, 2012; ISBN: 978-1451627916

Fighting Invisible Tigers: Stress Management for Teens

By Earl Hipp; Published by Free Spirit Publishing Inc., 2008; ISBN: 978-1575422824

Girls on the Edge: The Four Factors Driving the New Crisis for Girls—Sexual Identity, the Cyberbubble, Obsessions, Environmental Toxins

By Leonard Sax, MD, PhD; Published by Basic Books, 2010; ISBN: 978-0465015610

Just Between Us: A No-Stress, No-Rules Journal for Girls and Their Moms

By Meredith Jacobs and Sofie Jacobs; Published by Chronicle Books, 2010; ISBN: 978-0811868952

Living With Stress

By Allen R. Miller, PhD; Published by Checkmark Books, 2010; ISBN: 978-0816078882

Managing Stress: A Creative Journal

By Brian Luke Seaward; Published by Jones and Bartlett Publishers, 2004; ISBN: 978-0763723781

Marni: My True Story of Stress, Hair-Pulling, and Other Obsessions

By Marni Bates; Published by HCI Teens, 2009

My Anxious Mind: A Teen's Guide to Managing Anxiety and Panic

By Michael A. Tompkins, PhD and Katherine A. Martinez, PsyD; Published by Magination Press, 2009; ISBN: 978-1433804502

Posttraumatic Stress Disorder: Malady or Myth?
By Chris R. Brewin; Published by Yale University Press, 2007;
ISBN: 978-0300123746

The PTSD Workbook for Teens: Simple, Effective Skills for Healing Trauma
By Libbi Palmer, PsyD; Published by Instant Help, 2012; ISBN: 978-1608823215

Pressure: True Stories by Teens About Stress (Real Teen Voices Series)
By Youth Communication and Al Desetta, MA; Published by Free Spirit Publishing, 2012;
ISBN: 978-1575424125

Re-Defining Stress to Prevent Disease: Changing Thoughts, Perceptions, and Learned Experiences for Improved Health
By Steven Jaffe; Published by The Mind Diet Group, Inc., 2006; ISBN: 978-0972060585

The Stress Effect
By Richard Weinstein, DC; Published by Penguin Group (USA) Inc., 2004;
ISBN: 1583331816

Stress Free for Good: 10 Scientifically Proven Life Skills for Health and Happiness
By Dr. Frederic Luskin and Dr. Kenneth R. Pelletier; Published by HarperCollins Publishers,
Inc., 2005; ISBN: 006058274X

Stress 101: An Overview for Teens
By Margaret O. Hyde and Elizabeth H. Forsyth, MD; Published by Twenty-First Century
Books, 2007; ISBN: 978-0822567882

The Stress Reduction Workbook for Teens: Mindfulness Skills to Help You Deal With Stress; Published by Instant Help, 2010
By Gina M. Biegel; ISBN: 978-1572246973

Stress Relief: Ultimate Teen Guide
By Mark Powell; Published by The Scarecrow Press, 2007;
ISBN: 978-0810858060

Teen Stress Workbook

By John J Liptak, EdD and Ester A Leutenberg; Published by Whole Person Associates, 2011; ISBN: 978-1570252587

10 Simple Solutions to Stress:
How to Tame Tension and Start Enjoying Your Life

By Claire Michaels Wheeler, MD, PhD; Published by New Harbinger Publications, Inc., 2007; ISBN: 978-1572244764

Think Confident, Be Confident for Teens:
A Cognitive Therapy Guide to Overcoming
Self-Doubt and Creating Unshakable Self-Esteem

By Marci Fox, PhD and Leslie Sokol, PhD; Published by Instant Help, 2011; ISBN: 978-1608821136

Too Stressed to Think?
A Teen Guide to Staying Sane When Life Makes You Crazy

By Annie Fox and Ruth Kirschner; Published by Free Spirit Publishing, 2005; ISBN: 978-1575421735

Turn Stress into Bliss:
The Proven 8-Week Program for Health, Relaxation,
and Stress Relief

By Michael Lee; Published by Fair Winds Press, 2005; ISBN: 978-1592331178

Articles

"Academic Performance Top Cause of Teen Stress" from the Associated Press, accessed April 15, 2013, http://www.nbcnews.com/id/20322801/ns/health-childrens_health/t/academic -performance-top-cause-teen-stress/#.UWxPN7XqmSp.

"The Best Strategy for Reducing Stress" by Peter Bregman, *Harvard Business Review*, July 10, 2012, accessed April 15, 2013, http://blogs.hbr.org/bregman/2012/07/the-best-strategy-for -reducing.html.

"The Brain: 6 Lessons for Handling Stress" by Christine Gorman, *Time*, January 19, 2007, accessed April 15, 2013, http://www.time.com/time/magazine/article/0,9171,1580401-1,00.html.

"Bullies Are More Likely to Partake," *USA Today (Student Edition)*, April 2012, p. 15, accessed April 15, 2013, http://go.galegroup.com/ps/i.do?id=GALE%7CA286970612&v=2.1&u=cps15 40&it=r&inPS=true&prodId=GPS&userGroupName=cps1540&p=GPS&digest=db931a728 62d269de0699465b7ae7c6d&rssr=rss.

"Busy Bodies: Is Your Life So Hectic That You Can't Remember What Day of the Week It Is? If So, It May Be Time to Slow Things Down," by Leah Paulos, *Scholastic Choices*, November–December 2007, p. 6(6).

"Coping with Stress Holistically" by Lucia Thornton RN, MSN, AHN-BC, *Beginnings*, Winter 2010, pp. 16–19, accessed April 15, 2013, http://luciathornton.com/assets/files/Thornton _%20Beginnings_Winter2010_web%20edited%20final.pdf.

"Crisis in the Cafeteria (And We Don't Mean the Food)," by Elizabeth Foy Larsen, *Scholastic Choices*, January 2013, p. 9.

"Early Stress May Sensitize Girls' Brains for Later Anxiety," *Psychology & Sociology*, November 11, 2012, accessed April 15, 2013, http://esciencenews.com/articles/2012/11/11/early.stress.may .sensitize.girls.brains.later.anxiety.

"Good Stress" by Melinda Wenner, *Women's Health*, September 2009.

"Increased Stress Puts More at Risk (Teenagers)," *USA Today*, April 1, 2012, accessed April 15, 2013, http://www.accessmylibrary.com/article-1G1-286970570/increased-stress-puts-more.html.

"Infant Stress Affects Teen Brain" by Virginia Hughes, *Nature*, November 11, 2011, accessed April 15, 2013, http://www.nature.com/news/infant-stress-affects-teen-brain-1.11786.

"Peace of Mind: If You Always Feel Anxious and Stressed, You May Have Generalized Anxiety Disorder. Here's How to Reclaim a Sense of Calm," by Ben Kallen, *Natural Health*, December 2007, p. 57(5).

"RFV It Up: Feeling Fried? We've Got Super Simple Ways to Get Your Ooomph Back—No Red Bull Needed!" by Kara Wahlgren, *Girls' Life*, October–November 2007, p. 84(2).

"6 Lessons for Handling Stress," by Christine Gorman, *Time*, January 29, 2007, p. 80.

"Stress!?!" by Mackenzie Birkey, *Skipping Stones*, September–October 2007, p. 24(1).

"Stress Management is Easier for Empathetic Children" by Grace Rattue, *Medical News Today*, August 8, 2012, accessed April 15, 2013, http://www.medicalnewstoday.com/articles/248776.php.

"Stressed Out?" by Sara Rowe, *Boys' Life*, November 2011, 101(11) p. 36.

"Symptoms of Stress in Children," *Health*, April 10, 2013, accessed April 15, 2013, http://healthmagazine.ae/symptoms-of-stress-in-children.

"Teen Stress: How Much is Too Much?" by Raychelle Cassada Lohmann, MS, LPC, *Psychology Today*, September 30, 2011, accessed April 15, 2013, http://www.psychologytoday.com/blog/teen-angst/201109/teen-stress-how-much-is-too-much.

"Top Tips to Avoid School-Related Stress," *Health*, December 10, 2012, accessed April 15, 2013, http://healthmagazine.ae/top-tips-to-avoid-school-related-stress-2.

"When Sleep Becomes a Nightmare" by Matthew Hutson, *Scholastic Choices*, March 2013, p. 5.

Index

Index

Page numbers that appear in *Italics* refer to tables or illustrations. Page numbers that have a small 'n' after the page number refer to citation information shown as Notes. Page numbers that appear in **Bold** refer to information contained in boxes within the chapters.

A